Modern Living Kit
Health and Fitness

Modern Living Kit
Health and Fitness

Sudhanshu Shekhar Roy
Ravindranath Roy

AUTHORSPRESS

First Published 2001
by Authorspress

E-35/103, Jawahar Park,
Laxmi Nagar, Delhi-110 092

e-mail: authorspress@yahoo.com
quantum_soul@mantramail.com

Typeset in NewCenturySchlbk by Chitra Computers

Modern Living Kit: Health and Fitness
ISBN 81-7273-080-2

Printed in India at Mehra Offset Press, Delhi.

Preface

Health and fitness is not a static state—it is dynamic, ever-changing. Awareness about health and fitness is greater now than ever before, and the means to protect it available. Today, there is a growing emphasis on looking good, feeling good and living longer. Increasingly, scientific evidence tells us that one of the keys to achieving these ideals is fitness and exercise. Physical health is possible only through exercise and mental health through regulating our living in every facet of life. Regardless of age, gender or role in life, one can benefit from regular physical activity. If we are committed, exercise in combination with a sensible diet can help provide an overall sense of well-being and can even help prevent chronic illness, disability and premature death.

With the start of a new century, it is clear that fitness facilities must offer a variety of exercise options to meet the needs and lifestyles of a diverse population. Even in this age of fat-free and low-fat foods, our population continues to suffer from obesity. One explanation for this is that we are burning off fewer calories than we consume. This should come as no surprise as we look at our modern lifestyle, with its over-reliance on automobiles, computers and remote controls; all these items contribute to the sedentary living that has become so counterproductive to good health. Motivating this inactive population to incorporate regular exercise into their lives is the greatest challenge facing fitness professionals today. Health is not a commodity to be purchased in the market. It has to be earned the hard way, by getting every cell in our body under our control. There is no magical elixir to maintain fitness.

We should develop a certain honesty and practical approach to the problems of living, a good routine of daily exercise, and the right food. We must know the limits of our body and should not push it too far. Children should be trained right from a young age to think along correct lines for the attainment of health.

The book *Modern Living Kit: Health and Fitness* is intended to make people aware about how to keep good physical and mental health. It provides interesting information about health problems and physical activity programmes suitable for people from different age groups. The value of yoga in this fast moving age and stressed life is emphasised in this book. It will be an invaluable guide to all who are seeking alternative approaches to personal health, stress management, and mental health.

Authors

Contents

1

Effective Physical Fitness

Every day, we are inundated with health advertisements from the media, health professionals and well-intentioned friends and relatives. Most consumers are aware of the seemingly endless array of physical concerns associated with lifestyle and diet, and the implied promise of glowing good health and extended life, with the help of various healthcare programmes.

A healthy lifestyle is not defined solely by the food on one's plate. Meals with friends and family, enjoying traditional foods, sampling the cuisines of other cultures, and incorporating physical activity into a regular routine are all part of a healthful way of life. We have come a long way in our health and fitness knowledge. We know that an apple a day doesn't necessarily keep the doctor away and that a walk around the block once a week is not enough to keep fit.

Total health comprises of both mental and physical well-being. Your lifestyle determines your fitness consciousness, the will to keep fit or the ignorance which would ruins your health. The stress of the world today requires a striking balance between your physical fitness and your mental well-being for ensuring success without physical harm or degeneration.

Fitness is very personal. What is fit for your friend may not necessarily be fit for you. Age, sex, and heredity are all factors affecting fitness that you have no control over. You can improve the quality of your life by changing your personal habits, exercise routine, and eating behaviour.

Physical fitness means energetically performing daily tasks to the best of your ability without getting exhausted. Being physically fit also means that you still have energy to do the fun stuff that you love so much. You will be able to work hard and party hard, too, because all work and no play makes a person stressed, burnt-out, and very boring! You won't get sick as often because your immune system will be stronger. When you do get sick, you will recover faster and hopefully your symptoms won't be too gross.

Mental health means accepting all parts of you and being your own best friend. You don't beat yourself up over the things you can't control. Mental giants know when they are in over their heads and they concentrate on finding help. When high pressure situations pop up you won't stress and freak out; you will be able to deal because you are in complete control of your actions and reactions! You will be enjoying with the punches.

Being mentally strong means being positive and building support groups with friends who make you feel good about yourself and who give you a mental upbeat/high. You set goals and construct plans to achieve them. You don't need to cut other people down to feel good about yourself, so don't hang around with people who only feel good when they are cutting you down.

Getting fit will take time. You can start to develop your mental health by setting some realistic goals for yourself. Stop comparing your body with other people's bodies. This step is a doozie, so brace yourself—unless you are Aishwarya Rai or Amitabh Bachchan. When you think about it, this is really not a bad thing. You are absolutely unique.

Your genetic make-up is the blueprint for your body; genes determine lots of stuff—like whether or not you are going to have washboard abs or big boobs. Even if you do gazillion sit-ups and push-ups each day, your body is going to be programmed for washboard abs and big boobs before you can have them. That is why there are WonderBras and plastic surgery. We feel your pain, so here comes the good part: now that you have accepted the things you cannot change, you can change the things that you do have control over; to a point, anyway. There's always room for improvement, something you can change—even just little things that go a long way, like your attitude.

ESSENTIAL TIPS FOR PHYSICALLY ACTIVE

People who do not get enough physical activity are much more likely to develop heart diseases and high blood pressure. To maintain fitness and health one should start a physical activity programme, with the advice of a doctor.

Vigorous physical activity lowers an individual's risk of:

a) heart diseases and heart attack;
b) high blood pressure;
c) high cholesterol; and
d) high level of mental pressure.

If an individual has not been active and want to start exercising, first check with his/her doctor for a programme that is right for him/her. Once exercising is started, it would be realised that it is good for health and great fun also.

Physical activity should be enjoyable and can:

a) reduce chance of heart attack;
b) strengthen heart, lungs, bones and muscles;
c) give more energy and strength;
d) help to control weight and blood pressure;
e) help to handle stress;
f) help to sleep better; and
g) help to look good.

To help the heart, activities should be constant and lastlong enough to increase the blood-flow to the muscles. Start slowly and buildup as the heart gets stronger. First, the programme of exercise should be discussed with the doctor. Then try walking or hiking, jogging, bicycling, swimming, walking on a treadmill, stair climbing, aerobic dancing, cross-country skiing and so on.

In addition to exercise, easy-to-do daily activities may benefit the heart. Also, making small changes in the lifestyle can make a big overall difference in the health. Here are some examples:

a) Take a walk in the neighbourhood.
b) Get into gardening or yard work.
c) Take stairs instead of escalators and elevators.
d) Park farther from store and walk through the parking lot.
e) Learn a new dance/sport.
f) Talk to your doctor, or healthcare professional.
g) If one has heart disease, members of the family also may be at higher risk. It is very important for them to make changes now to lower their risk.
h) Take few minutes to write your own questions for the next time you see your doctor. For example:
i) What is the best type of exercise for me?
j) How much should I exercise?
k) What do I exercise ?
l) What do I eat?

A regular exercise programme helps to:

a) reduce the risk of heart disease by improving blood circulation throughout the body.
b) Keep weight under control.
c) Improve blood cholesterol levels.
d) Prevent and manage high blood pressure.
e) prevent bone loss.

f) Boost energy level.

g) Help to manage stress.

h) release tension.

i) improve the ability to fall asleep quickly and sleep well.

j) Improve self image.

k) counter anxiety and depression and increases enthusiasm and optimism.

l) Increase muscle strength, give greater capacity for other physical activities.

m) provide a way to share an activity with family and friends.

n) Establish good heart-healthy habits in children and counters the conditions that led to heart attack and stroke later in life.

o) Prevent chronic illnesses and diseases associated with aging and maintains quality of life and independence later.

Importance of Walking

Try a walk, if you feel sluggish or drained. Walking is more than just a way to keep your heart healthy. It is a whole new way of life. It helps you meet people. It boosts your energy. It will help you to take control of your life and health. It encourages you to make walking a way of life.

Walking can be an aerobic exercise that conditions your heart and lungs. It is best to walk at vigorous intensity for 30-60 minutes three or four times a week. But even low- to moderate- intensity walking can have both short- and long-term benefits. If done daily, you can help lower your risk of heart disease.

On the other hand, physical inactivity is a risk factor for heart disease. Combined with overeating, lack of exercise may lead to high blood cholesterol, obesity, high blood pressure and even diabetes, which are all risk factors for heart disease.

To lose weight, you can eat your usual amount of calories, but exercise more. For example, a 100 kg. person who eats the same amount of calories but walks briskly each day for 11/2 miles could lose about 7 kg. in one year.

Besides helping you to control your weight, walking may:

a) help to avoid cigarette smoking;
b) help to control blood pressure; and
c) help to raise your HDL, or good cholesterol level.

Aerobic exercise may not prevent or cure heart disease. But it is a positive step towards a healthier life. Besides cardiovascular benefits, a regular physical activity like walking gives you more energy, improves your self-image, increases resistance to fatigue, helps you to relax and feel less tense, and increases the ability to fall asleep quickly and sleep well.

When you are ready to start a regular, vigorous walking programme, you may want to see your doctor first. You definitely should seek medical advice if:

a) your doctor said you have a heart condition and recommended only medically supervised physical activity.
b) during or right after you exercise, you frequently have pains or pressure in the left or mid-chest area, left neck, shoulder or arm.
c) you have developed chest pain within the last month.
d) you tend to lose consciousness or fall over due to dizziness.
e) you feel extremely breathless after mild exertion.
f) your doctor recommended you take medicine for your blood pressure or a heart condition.
g) your doctor said you have bone or joint problems that could be made worse by the proposed physical activity.
h) you have a medical condition or other physical reason not mentioned here that might need special attention in an exercise programme.

i) you are middle-aged or older, have not been physically active, and plan a relatively vigorous exercise programme.

j) if none of these conditions apply to you, you can start gradually on a programme tailored to your needs, if you feel any.

k) in case of any discomfort while applying a programme, contact your doctor right away.

To ensure a successful walking programme, choose the best time for you. Then stick with a specific time. When do you have the most energy? Some people walk in the morning to get ready for the day. Some walk during lunch hour. Others walk toward the end of the day to relieve tension and relax.

Some people do not have a full 30-60 minutes to walk. That is all right. Recent research suggests that three 10-minute or two 15-minute periods provide about the same benefit as one 30-minute period. So try to accumulate a full 30-60 minutes by doing some combination of the following:

a) 10 to 15-minute walk during your breaks
b) 10 to 15-minute walk after meals.

You should have an annual calendar for exercise. So it is best to choose a place where you can walk all the time. For outdoor walking, find a course with a smooth, soft surface that does not intersect with traffic. When weather prevents outdoor walking, walk around an indoor track at a school or walk on a treatment or cycle on an exercise cycle or you could put on your walking shoes and walk around shopping malls. Regardless of where you walk, be sure it is well lighted.

It is all right to walk alone. But companions will make walking more enjoyable and help you stick to your programme, find some person/group to walk with you. Your walking partners should be able to keep the same schedule and walk the same pace as you. I suggest this from the living example my father who had a group of 'morning walkers', who have drawn from different professions walked together continuously for nearly 20 years. Any absence from the morning walk had to be explained to the members. The pressure of the group for walking was such that members rarely absented form their walking programme.

It is important to walk in the right kind of shoes. Choose shoes with thick, flexible soles that cushion the sole of the foot and absorb shock for the rest of the body.

If you walk outside, during the winter, layer your clothing to keep out the cold and wind. The best materials are cotton, fleece-lined cotton, wool or a breathable nylon. These materials allow sweat to evaporate and keep you warm and dry. Be sure to wear warm socks, a sweat-shirt with a hood or a hat, gloves and a turtle neck muffler to keep all areas of your body covered.

In the summer, wear cotton or other porous materials that will allow sweat to evaporate. Be sure to drink plenty of water before/after and during your walk when it is hot.

Warm up by walking slowly for about five minutes. After that, you can do stretching exercises. This will limber up your body and prepare it for more strenuous exercise. You can also do moderate exercises such as jumping rope.

Stretching exercises include:

a) *Wall push*: Stand one and a half feet away from a wall. Lean forward pushing against the wall with your hands, keeping your heels flat on the ground. Hold it for 10 seconds, then relax. Repeat once or twice.

b) *Palm touch*: Bend your knees slightly. Try to touch the floor by bending from the waist. Do not bounce. Hold the position for 10 seconds, then repeat once or twice. If you have lower back problems, do the same thing, but with your legs crossed.

c) *Toe touch*: Place your right leg on a chair or railing, making a 90-degree angle with the other leg. Keep the left leg straight and lean forward, touching the toes of the right leg. Again, do not bounce. Switch legs and do the same thing. Repeat the entire exercise once or twice.

d) *Fresh-ups*: Place both your hands on the floor with legs straight, supported by your toe bend your elbow and take 2-3 dips. Repeat once or twice after intervals without straining yourselves.

Set a pace for your programme and do not push yourself too hard when you start. Reduce your pace if:

a) you are unable to speak easily in a conversational tone;

b) it takes longer than five minutes for your pulse to slow down after you exercise; and

c) you feel faint, have a hard-time breathing or have prolonged weakness.

Try to do at least three exercise sessions a week. Each session should consist of a warm-up for about five minutes, an exercise period 30 to 60 minutes depending on where you are in your programme, and a five-minute cool down.

If you are ready to start walking, you may want to begin with the programme suggested below.

a) Walk briskly 5 min. to 15 min.

b) Walk briskly 7 min. to 17 min.

c) Walk briskly 9 min. to 19 min.

d) Walk briskly 11 min. to 21min

e) Walk briskly 13 min. to 23 min.

f) Walk briskly 15 min. to 25 min.

g) Walk briskly 18 min. to 28 min.

h) Walk briskly 20 min. to 30 min.

i) Walk briskly 23 min. to 33 min.

j) Walk briskly 26 min. to 36 min.

k) Walk briskly 28 min. to 38 min.

l) Walk briskly 30 min. to 40 min.

The figures below show the approximate calories per hour spent by a 75, 100, 150 or 200 pound person performing a particular activity.

Walking, 2 mph	125	160	240	320
Walking, 3 mph	175	210	320	420
Walking, 41/2 mph	245	295	440	590
Jogging, 51/2 mph	365	440	740	880
Jogging, 7 mph	510	610	920	1220

To calculate your resting heart rate take your heart rate on a regular basis right after you wakeup in the morning to ensure that you will have your real resting heart rate. Count how many beats per 10 seconds your heart will beat. By keeping track of your resting heart rate you will notice that as time goes on, and as you become fitter, your resting heart rate will lower. The average resting heart rate is 12-13 beats/10 seconds.

You can calculate your recovery heart rate by the following techniques.

Ten seconds immediately after you have finished the exercise, take a pulse check. Remember that number. Multiply that number by six. One minute after the first pulse check, take another pulse check and remember that number. Multiply that number by six. Whatever the difference is between the first pulse check you took and the second pulse check is your recovery heart rate. If the difference is bigger between the first and the second pulse check it means that you are in better shape.

To calculate your target rate zone, subtract your age from 220—so 220 your age (A). Whatever the difference is between 220 and your age (A), is your maximum heart rate (MHR) Multiply your MHR by 6.8 and divide whatever number you get by 6. This is the upper limit of your target heart rate zone in a 10 second count.

$$(A) \times 0.8 = b$$

b/6 = upper limit of target heart rate zone (Y)

Multiply your MHR by 0.6 and divide the resulting number by 6. This is the lower limit of your target heart rate zone in a 10 second count.

$$(A) \times 0.6 = c$$

$$c/6 = \text{lower limit of target heart rate zone (Z)}$$

So you target heart rate zone is between (Y) and (Z) beats per 10 seconds. Your maximum heart rate is the most your heart rate should reach after a strenuous workout. Checking one's heart rate is also known as taking a pulse check.

You can take a pulse rate by using two fingers (usually your index and middle finger—mind you never use your thumb). Press them lightly against the place where you are to take your pulse. If you use your thumb you can feel a different pulse and that pulse is going at a different rate than the other pulse points. You can take a pulse check at your carotid (the area on your neck below the jaw), your radial (on the wrist, the side of your thumb), your chest (the area that is just above your heart on your chest slightly to the side).

You can check your heart rate:

i) *After your warm-up:* Then your heart rate should be close to the lower end of your target zone. If you are up over by the upper limit of your target HR zone slow down the next time you do your warm-up.

ii) *Halfway into your workout*: If it is higher than the upper limit pull back and ease off on the intensity that you are working at.

iii) *At the end of your workout*: Your HR should be up there—if your HR is within the lower end of your zone work harder on your next workout.

iv) *At the end of your cool-down*: Your heart rate should be around your resting rate— if it is still up there then take a little more time just to walk around a bit and bring your heart rate down.

Keep moving while you are checking your heart rate—be it marching on the spot or a slower version of the movement you were doing before the HR check this is to ensure that you get a reasonable reading for your heart rate and that you don't lose track of the 10 second count.

Factors affecting heart rate includes:

a) *Emotions*: When you are feeling stressed your heart rate will jump by a significant number are, i.e., your heart starts racing whenever you see that special someone or your heart races when you realise you forgot to study for that mid-term test.

b) *Temperature*: If you are working out in a hot climate or have a fever your heart rate will naturally be higher because it is working to supply oxygen to your muscles and body.

c) *Posture*: When you are lying down your heart rate is slower than if you were to sit up. Your heart rate when you are standing is higher that your HR when you are sitting. More energy is required of the body to stand than to lie down.

d) *Size*: The heart rate for a person who carries more weight than the usual weight for that person will have a higher heart rate in order to supply energy to the body.

Make Physical Activity a Way of Life

If one is not in the habit of being physically active, it is better to start a physical exercise programme. Because a physical activity programme help to reduce some dangerous risk factors like high blood pressure when they are physically active. Vigorous activity on a regular basis also can help lose weight and reduce cholesterol level, two other risk factors for heart disease. Some major guidelines maintain a successful physical activity programme are given below.

a) Talk to your doctor about activities that are right for you.

b) Choose a starting date that fits your schedule which gives you enough time to begin your programme.

c) Wear comfortable clothes and shoes.

d) Try to exercise at the same time of day so it becomes a regular part of your lifestyle.

e) Drink a cup of water before, during and after activity periods greater that 30 minutes in length.

f) Ask a friend to start a programme with you —use buddy system.

g) Note your activities on a calendar. Write down the distance or length of time you workout and how you fell after each session.

h) If you miss a day, plan a make-up day or add 10-15 minutes to your next session.

i) Get your family to participate in fun activities. It is great to have a support system, and you will be getting them into an important health habit.

j) Choose activities you like and make sure they are convenient for you. If you need a good weather, have a backup plan for bad days (e.g., when it rains, walk in the mall instead of the park).

k) Learn a new sport you think you might enjoy, or take lesson to improve atone you know.

l) Use variety to keep your interest up. Walk one day, take a swim the next time you exercise, then go for a bike-ride on the weekend.

m) Get yourself in a regular routine so being physically active becomes a habit that you do automatically.

n) If you stop for any length of time, do not lose hope. Just get started again gradually and work-up to your old pace.

o) Try not to compare yourself with others. Your goal should be enjoyment and personnel fitness.

p) Do not quit if you miss a week. Remind yourself of all the reason you started.

q) Do not push yourself too hard. You should be able to talk during exercise.

r) If you have heart disease, members of your family also may be at higher risk. It is very important for them to make changes now to lower their risk.

s) Take a few minutes to write your own question for the next time you seen your doctor, fore example:

t) Should I take my pulse?

u) Can I exercise too much ?

v) Can I jog (body weight may be taken into consideration)?

w) What should be the weight training I do?

REFERENCES

Bud Getchell Alan E. Mikesky Kay Mikesky, *Physical Fitness: A Way of Life*, 1998.

Cooper, Robert K., *Health And Fitness Excellence*, Boston: Houghton Mifflin, 1989.

Daniel Girdano, Dorothy E. Dusek George S. Everly, *Controlling Stress and Tension*, 2001.

Darden, Ellington, *Living Longer Stronger*, New York: Burkley Publishing, 1995.

David K. Miller T. Earl Allen, *Fitness: A Lifetime Commitment*, 1995.

Hoeger, Werner and Sharon Hoeger, *Lifetime Physical Fitness And Wellness*, Englewood, CO: Morton Publishing, 1992.

Jerrold S. Greenberg George B. Dintiman Barbee Myers Oakes, *Wellness: Creating a Life of Health and Fitness*, 1997.

Larry Brown, H., *Lifetime Fitness*, 1996.

On The Run: Exercise And Fitness For Busy People, Waitz, Grete Paperback ISBN: 1579542530.

Optimum Health For The New Millennium, Townsend, Ernestine Paperback ISBN: 0738837970.

Richard Polidoro J., *Sport and Physical Activity in the Modern World*, 2000.

Robert W. Buckingham Ph.D., *Primer on International Health*, 2001.

Sally A. Althoff Milan Svoboda Daniel Girdano, *Choices in Wellness for Life*, 1996.

2

Nutrition for Fitness

Nutrition plays a vital role in maintaining mental and physical fitness. It has a major impact on heart health and physical fitness. Your body needs food for fuel. Like a car, your body won't work well if you do not have a well-balanced mix of fuel. Physical activity can decrease risk factors linked with coronary heart disease; help improve your ability to exercise and do physical work; increase enthusiasm and foster a sense of well-being; release tension and help you relax and sleep; help control your weight; and encourage positive changes in other lifestyle habits. Good eating habits are the key in helping you achieve these goals.

The nutritional needs of human beings vary from person to person. Basically, there are three genetic metabolic types of bodies among human beings: ectomorph, endomorph and mesomorph. Some of us gain weight with difficulty, some of us put on fat easily and some of us put on muscle watching television. The genetic differences between individuals is great. Body type has little to do with athletic ability or coordination, it simply relates to metabolism and genetic predisposition to gaining fat or muscle or staying lean. Athletic ability and coordination are also tied to genetics but not the body type/ metabolism genes.

Ectomorphs generally have a very high metabolic rate making it difficult for the to gain both muscle and fat. They are naturally lean individuals. They need less aerobics and should do anaerobic/strength building resistance training with reps in the six to 10 range.

Mesomorphs are the guys who can come into the gym only occasionally but stay lean and pack on muscle very easily. Some mesomorphs are muscular, defined and have 'six pack abs' with little or no exercise. Probably most professional body builders are mesomorphs.

Endomorphs are people who tend to put on fat. They tend to have a lower metabolic rate. They need to do more aerobics and higher rep, 12-20 reps, anaerobics in order to burn more calories. Adding muscle through anaerobic exercise will increase the basal metabolic rate. Please do not make these categories strict 'pigeon holes' to put yourself or workout partners in. Ultimately the ectomorph has little mesomorph in him/her. The endomorph also has a little mesomorph in him/her. It is just that some of us work a little harder to bring out the mesomorph.

The amount and type of exercise required by each of us is different. This synergistic exercise programme is adaptable to all three body types. We all need aerobic exercise, however lean. People obviously need less aerobics than heavy people. No matter what your body type the Ultimate Aerobic and Anaerobic Programme will provide an excellent total body workout or an excellent warm up for your specific exercise programme. The combination of lower body aerobics and upper body aerobics provides muscle stimulation with the resultant increased nutrient and oxygen rich blood flow to all the muscles of your body.

To ectomorphs some aerobics (20 minutes, three times per week minimum) are required for cardiovascular fitness—low rep 6-10 with heavier weights to gain size—longer rest between sets, two-three minutes. If a ectomorph's goal includes optimal physical condition, he needs more aerobics. For optimal cardiovascular fitness aerobic conditioning is required.

Mesomorphs need aerobics for cardiovascular fitness (20 minutes, three times per week minimum); a balanced programme of low rep for size and high rep for definition. If a mesomorph's goal includes optimal physical condition, he needs more aerobics. For optimal cardiovascular fitness aerobic conditioning is required.

Endomorphs need lots of aerobics to burn calories/fat (30-40 minutes, three-five times per week); higher rep 12-20 with lower weights and short rest intervals, 30-60 seconds between sets.

This professionally designed synergistic exercise programme systematically exercises all the major muscle groups of the body in a thorough aerobic and anaerobic/resistive fashion. Aerobics utilising the muscles of the upper body is equally as effective as aerobics for the muscles of the lower body for cardiovascular/endurance training. In activities of daily living upper body endurance and strength are every bit important, or even more, as lower body strength and endurance.

The participants in this aerobic exercise and strength building programme experience a complete cardiovascular workout, muscle toning, calorie burning, metabolic enhancement, posture improvements, body-shaping and weight-loss in one complete programme.

Current researches recommend strength building, anaerobic exercise combined with an aerobic exercise programme. According to the researches aerobic exercise is essential for weight loss, cardiovascular fitness and body-shaping. Anaerobic exercise is essential for strength building and muscle gain. Combining aerobic and anaerobic exercise is optimal. Benefits of the ultimate aerobic and anaerobic exercise is optimal. Benefits of the ultimate aerobic and anaerobic exercise programme include: improved endurance, strength, range from motion, balance, posture and coordination.

An anabolic and growth hormone-friendly diet should include plenty of animal protein, sufficient good fat and carbohydrates. Such a diet is anabolic and is appropriate for any healthy and active individual. If you have special medical dietary or conditions, you should consult your physician.

Eat sufficient protein, lots of vegetables and fruits and minimal processed carbohydrates. No magic, just intelligent, planned and scheduled nutrient consumption. In order to be compliant with the anti-aging and longevity project recommendations, nutrient consumption scheduling is necessary. Including sufficient protein and fat is anabolic, or conducive to tissue/muscle growth and hormonal secretions.

Animal protein can be got from lean beef, skinless chicken, eggs, fish, etc. Take protein 20-60 grams per day. Take good oils with in 20 per cent-30 per cent total calories. Specific essential fatty acids are needed for most of the body's hormonal functions. The oil must have the proper fatty acid composition and molecular bonding.

Some commonly available good oils are:

a) Flax oil: Supplement 3-6 grams of per day.
b) Omega-3 fish oils: Supplement 3-6 grams per day.
c) Olive or Canola oil for salads and cooking.
d) Trim the fat out of the beef and pull the skin off the chicken.
e) Raw fruits and vegetables are nutrient dense and fibre rich.
f) Processed grain are mostly useless, non nutritious calories with minimal fibre.

Metabolism and cellular replication are carried out by a number of processes including many components. The classes on nutrition were mixed with courses on microbiology, and anatomy and physiology provided credence to the principles of science in nutrition.

The microbiology and physiology of tissues at the cellular level documents the complex nature of providing the cells the needed raw materials through proper nutrition and supplementation. The exact nutrients necessary for optimum function change throughout the day.

Our hormonal and physiologic needs change with activity and time of day (circadian rhythms). This is why we offer different formulations of the secretagogue stacks depending on the time of the day and the situation. The nutrients necessary for cellular replication, hormonal secretions, and neural function are not random and unspecific. The numbers of specific nutrients that must be present in the body, simultaneously, and in the proper ratios is phenomenal for the millions of chemical reactions that are occurring constantly and simultaneously in our bodies 24 hours per day.

The last three decades were years of fad diets. The late 1970's saw the liquid high protein diets. Beginning in the 1980s the aversion to any kind of fat began. Then the high carbohydrate diet became the thing. None of these ever made any sense. But marketing and pop-media convinced millions of people that proper nutrition was unimportant and that fad diets were the way to go. As we are in the 21st century, science at the cellular level has changed and complicated much of the previous nutritional philosophy.

NUTRITIONAL LINKS

Some simple rules that can make food choices and proper nutrition easier:

a) The more unprocessed a food is the better. Corn on the cob is better than corn chips.

b) Dark green vegetables are better than light green vegetables. Broccoli is better than iceberg lettuce.

c) Broccoli carrots, tomatoes, spinach and some cauliflower make a nutrient packed vegetable salad combination.

d) Be careful with choices of meat.

e) Leaner cuts are better.

f) Pull the skin off the chicken and cut most of the fat out of the meat.

g) The current theory is that red meat is not our enemy. A natural source for the body-building supplement creating is red meat.

h) Fat is required for most hormonal secretions and functions.

i) Meat and eggs are generally complete proteins. They have all the essential amino acids but tend to have more fat, and less healthy fat, than vegetables. But again the current recommendations are for more dietary fat. However, there are friendlier fats than beef tallow.

j) Fish is always a good choice, especially cold water fish with their omega-3 fatty acids.

k) Beans have protein but are not complete proteins because they do not have all of the essential amino acids, but when combined with rice or corn become a complete protein. However both beans and grains are carbohydrates and in order to consume enough of these carbs to meet daily protein requirements would require a considerable volume of carbohydrates.

l) White bread and pastas are sugar's second cousin. The glycemic index principles cannot be taught here of how fast the glucose enters the bloodstream. But back to the process vs. unprocessed, brown rice is better than instant white rice, and whole wheat is better than processed grains (white bread or white, processed pasta).

m) Follow a diet heavy on dark coloured vegetables, unprocessed whole grains and lean meats, and you can not go wrong.

Obesity is the biggest health problem facing most of the urban population across the world. More than half of us are over our ideal weight and more than one-third are obese enough to significantly raise the risk of disease and premature death. Nutrition is one of the greatest weapons against diseases, keeping fats at about 20-30 per cent of caloric intake.

Eating five or more servings a day of fruit and vegetables lowers your chances of getting cancer.

The advocates of the low carbohydrate, ketogenic diet cringe at the thought of multi servings of fruit. However, moderation is a key to a stable life. Professional body-builders have different goals than a person eating for health. Persons with extreme weight loss requirements obviously have different needs than the average weight conscious person. Persons striving for a five per cent body fat and rippled abs probably also have different goals than simply enjoying a healthy life.

COOKING FOR GOOD NUTRITION

Choose methods of cooking that will retain flavour, colour and nutrients. Steam instead of boiling vegetables. Avoid cooking at high temperatures and long cooking times. Both extended heat and liquid can destroy or leach out valuable nutrients. Add vegetables whenever possible to ensure your five-a-day intake. Experiment with more vegetable variety in salads, try new vegetable mixes, include some shredded vegetables in casseroles, and add different vegetables to soups and stews.

Use chopped red or yellow peppers to 'pep-up' the flavour. Try vegetable salads and fruit chutneys as accompaniments to meat or poultry in place of heavy sauces. When you use oil, select olive, sunflower or canola oil. Drain off visible fat while cooking, blot pan-fried foods on paper towels to absorb extra grease. Hormones are secreted by the endocrine system and used at the cellar level for communication between body tissues including the brain, organs, other glands, muscles and other tissues of the body.

HORMONES AND NUTRITIONAL SUPPLEMENTATION

Hormones are secreted by the endocrine system and used at the cellular level for communication between body tissues including the brain, organs, other glands, muscles and other tissues of the body. There are two types of glands that compose the endocrine system:

a) exocrine glands and
b) endocrine glands.

The exocrine glands secrete their hormones into ducts and body cavities. The glands include sweat glands, oil glands, and digestive glands. The endocrine glands secrete into capillaries to be transported with the blood. These glands release hormones into the bloodstream.

The endocrine glands include the pituitary, thyroid, parathyroid, adrenals, pineal, thymus, and hypothalamus. In addition there are organs of the body which contain the endocrine tissue but that are not exclusively endocrine glands such as the pancreas, ovaries, testes, kidneys, stomach, skin and heart. These hormones, glandular secretions, control many of our short-term and long-term bodily functions.

Although hormones are chemically diverse they are constructed from amino acids and cholesterol. They can be divided into three classes:

a) amines,
b) proteins and peptides, and
c) steroids.

Amines are the simplest hormone molecules and are fabricated from amino acids. These hormones are extremely important in metabolism and energy production.

Proteins and peptides are long chains of amino acids and are large molecules. Insulin secreted by the pancreas is an example.

Steroids are hormones fabricated from cholesterol. Examples include aldosterone, testosterone and estrogen.

Our growth, mood, digestion, respiration, sense of thirst and hunger, sexual functions, fat metabolism and most other bodily functions are all triggered by hormones. The amount of hormone released or secreted by the endocrine glands is determined by the body's need for that particular hormone at a given time. Once the hormone is secreted into the circulatory system it is transported by the blood to all areas of the body but only specific target cells react to their presence.

Target cells contain receptors that respond to specific hormones being transported throughout the body by the circulatory system. There are thousands of receptors in each of our cells. Each of these receptors responds to a specific hormone's unique amino acid chain or pattern. Once the hormone is bound to the receptor cell a chain of genetically predetermined biochemical events within the target cell occur.

The degree to which the target cell responds to the hormone depends on the number of target cells, genetics and the concentration of the hormone. In effect, the amino acid structure of the hormone is the key and the receptor is a lock. In order for the key, hormone, to fit the lock receptor, the hormone-receptor complex must be an exact match. If for any reason this lock and key do not fit, the cellular binding is disrupted, the hormonal signals are interrupted and the communication is not complete.

Hormones also interact with other hormones to price-specific metabolic responses. In some cases the effect is synergistic, that is, the cellular response is more than the sum of hormones involved (1 + 1 + 1 = 4), they compliment each other. In some cases the effect is antagonistic, one hormone stops or reduces the action of another hormone (1 + 1 = 0).

A natural and expected effect of aging is the decrease in function and effectiveness of body structures and tissues. The most obvious are our skin and eyesight. Glandular function, metabolic function, endocrine system function, immune system function, proteins synthesis, protein assimilation and most other body functions are similarly affected by aging. The effect of this is that the endocrine systems, functional demise can be compared to the 'chemical telephone lines' being down. The various parts of the body do not properly communicate with each other. The intracellular and intercellular chemical instructions are interrupted and body parts in effect become hormonally isolated from one another. Messages that would normally prompt cellular rejuvenation are never sent or received. Consequently, cells grow old, losing natural healthiness.

As we become old, most of our glands secrete less and less of the hormone they are designed to secrete. There are times when the regulatory systems do not operate properly. As we age this regulation becomes less efficient and hormone levels change. The amount of hormones released by the endocrine glands is determined by the bodies needs for the hormones at a given time.

However, the endocrine glands can be stimulated to release more hormones, more frequently. A remarkable amount of data has been compiled that indicates that many of the 'diseases' that the middle-aged begin experiencing, including depression, poor sleep, abdominal weight gain, muscle loss as well as prostate and heart conditions are directly related to hormone/ endocrine/glandular imbalances that can be correct with currently available medication and nutritional therapies.

Replacing the hormones which decline with age is as important to the treatment of aging as is replacing normal levels of insulin is to an insulin-dependent diabetic. Women have seen a dramatic reduction in the infirmities of aging, general health improvements, with the increased use of the hormone estrogen as a safe and effective Hormone Replacement Therapy.

The Human Growth Hormone (HGH) secreted by the anterior pituitary responding to chemical, hormonal instructions from the hypothalamus, is composed of over 190 amino acids arranged in a particular order or chain. If any of these amino acids are not present at the correct position in the chain it is not HGH. If any these amino acids are not present proper cellular binding will not occur.

The endocrine system is composed of a complex network of glands that secrete hormones. Hormones are in effect the chemical messengers of the body. These hormones are essential for the regulation of many of our biological processes. These are the chemical messengers of our body. Our sense of thirst, hunger, mood, immune system, sexual function, growth pattern and most other biological functions are dependent on the appropriate levels of hormonal secretions by a variety of glands often working in conjunction with each other.

There are 22 essential and non essential amino acids which are fabricated into something like 50,000 proteins. All amino acids can be fabricated from the eight essential amino acids. Some textbooks state that there are conditional amino acids that the body cannot synthesise under certain conditions. Current research indicates that the anterior pituitary can be stimulated with nutritional supplementation and exercise to increase the HGH secretion, and the adrenals can be stimulated to produce more hormones, as can the thyroid and the pancreas.

The anterior pituitary under chemical/hormonal instructions from the hypothalamus produces HGH. HGH blood levels diminish after adolescence, the measured levels decline each decade of our life. HGH is produced throughout our lives but the blood levels go down. Many of the effects associated with aging are associated with declining HGH levels such as thin skin and skin wrinkles; muscle wasting; abdominal fat; cognitive changes; mood changes; decreasing energy; sexual performance; weak bones; reduced cardiac output, and so on.

These conditions are directly or indirectly affected by the decline in HGH levels present in our system. HGH is critical for tissue repair, brain function, physical health, mental health, muscle growth, bone strength, energy, and any other cellular functions. This decline in HGH level is not irreversible.

If you are in your 30s you can stimulate growth hormone release and keep your body supplies from decreasing. If you are in your 40s, 50s, 60s or older there are nutritional programmes to recharge our dwindling supply. If for some reason your body has completely stopped producing HGH, then there is replacement hormone therapy, actual HGH injections.

The three methods of raising the systemic levels of HGH are:

a) Recombinant HGH and cadaver HGH are available by prescription for injection.
b) Manipulating HGH production by the anterior pituitary through specific amino acid and nutrient supplementation combinations.
c) Exercise.

The anterior pituitary reacts to specific amino acids and nutrient combinations by increasing production of HGH. The hypothalamus and the pituitary in conjunction stimulate HGH production based on other factors. There are many commercial products available that profess to increase HGH levels.

HGH is at its peak during adolescence. It continued to be produced throughout our lives, however in increasingly diminished amounts. The fact that HGH production is reduced significantly as we age is a major factor in aging. HGH is critical for tissue repair, healing, brain function, physical health, mental health, muscle growth, bone strength, energy and metabolism, and its demise is a major factor in aging. As you can see many of the effects of aging are controlled by the HGH.

HGH Synergy

Blood levels of HGH can be increased by three ways:

a) Non-prescription supplementation of amino acid secretagogues and dietary control.
b) Exercise, hard aerobics and moderate anaerobics. Exercise stimulates HGH production.
c) Prescription rHGH. Actual HGH via injection requires a doctors' prescription.

The anti-aging and longevity project's focus has been on the manipulation of HGH secretion and systemic blood levels through oral supplementation and synergistic exercise.

a) Raising levels of HGH through supplementation is well documented.
b) Raising HGH through exercise is also well documented.
c) Exercises are synergistic.

Increasing growth hormone levels through supplementation enables one to:

a) burn more fat;
b) increase muscle mass;
c) improve immune function; and
d) increase skin thickness

The list of exercise benefits is parallel to the effects of growth hormone stimulation. Persons who participate in a regular exercise programme will experience:

a) increased growth hormone secretion.

b) fat loss.

c) increased muscle mass and strength.

d) improvement in immune response.

e) extended and improved lifespan

Combining nutritional supplementation with synergistic exercises puts a double whammy on fat and aging. Controlling hormone levels is the best way to improve both body composition and to slowdown aging. Hormone levels can be controlled through dietary supplementation of amino acid secretagogues, exercises and prescription medications. Growth hormone promotes and increases in the synthesis of new protein tissue and retards the breakdown of protein tissue that can occur with dietary deficiencies, exercise stress or other factors.

Although growth hormone has powerful protein building effect it is probably more potent in its ability to promote the breakdown of stored body fat. Growth hormone not only stimulates body and muscle growth directly, it also stimulates the body's production of other anabolic growth factors circulating in the bloodstream. The most powerful of these other hormones are the insulin-like growth factors. In addition to stimulating the insulin-like growth factors, the HGH interacts with these hormones in such a way that the net effect of all of them is to produce a reduction in fat tissue while increasing lean tissue/muscle mass.

If we consider aging a disease and not just a normal occurrence, it follows that anyone who wants to maintain his youthful vigour and endurance should include an effective growth hormone stimulation therapy as part of his health regiment. One study conducted by Ralph Paffenbarger and his colleagues involving 17,000 Harvard alumni found that men who burned 500 to 1,000 calories a week on physical activity had a 22 per cent lower risk of death for all causes, while those who expended 2,500 calories a week also added one to two years to their extended lifespan.

People who are physically fit, eat a healthy, balanced diet and take nutritional supplements can slice 10 to 20 years off their biological age—the true age that your body should be measured, in terms of function, rather than your chronological age as measured by the candles on your birthday cake.

The two hormones that men are most concerned with are HGH and testosterone. Women have been getting oestrogen replacement therapy as an acceptable Medical Hormone Replacement Therapy for decades. HGH replacement therapy is more effective when used together with DHEA and other hormones. Estrogen/progesterone replacement for women or testosterone replacement for men can also add significantly to benefits from hormone replacement.

The goal of hormone replacement is to restore levels to those normally present for several decades during early adulthood. The safe levels at age 30 will remain safe when restored to that same level later in life. Adverse effects from hormone replacement result only from excessive doses or the use of unnatural and synthetic hormones.

Control of Hormonal Secretions

Hormonal secretions are the basic components in the communication process of the endocrine system. The secretions are composed of amino acids. Through supplementation of specific amino acids at specific times we can have a great effect, in effect, manipulate the hormonal system. Specific glands use specific and unique combinations of amino acids and nutrients to trigger specific responses and glandular/hormonal secretions. By combining specific amino acids and other nutrients we can trigger desired responses to specific glands.

Some of the human functions affected by HGH include:

a) fat metabolism

b) muscle growth

c) sexual performance

d) organ function

e) cardiac output

f) stronger bones

g) faster healing

h) younger skin and wrinkle reduction

i) mood elevation

j) cognitive improvement.

ROLE OF AMINO ACIDS IN NUTRITION

Amino acids used in the secretagogue stacks are identical to the amino acids present in food. Proteins are composed of amino acids. Egg protein, beef protein, milk protein and soy protein all have different amino acid ratios and composition. In order for the amino acids to be used by the body as protein, all the required amino acids must be present in the gut at the same time. This is the concept of combining beans and rice for a complete protein is based on the fact that all eight essential amino acids must be present at the same time. For a complete protein to be formed is integral to the timing of amino acid secretagogue supplementation. If the secretagogues are present with the essential amino acids the secretagogues will be used as protein instead of HGH releasing secretagogues.

In human body, there are eight essential amino acids and 14 non-essential amino acids that can be fabricated from the eight essential amino acids. From these 22 amino acids, being combined and arranged into varying specific chains, all proteins are fabricated by the human body. These are the basic building blocks that combine into literally thousands of complex protein, amino acid chains.

Amino acids are organic compounds with at least one amino group and one carboxyl group. The amino groups include at least one NH_3 molecule. The carboxyl contains at least one COOH molecule. These molecules are combined in long chains to form proteins.

Amino acids are necessary for endocrine secretions, enzymes, components of structure and elements of the immune system. They are precursors to many important micro-molecules such as dopamine, epinephrine, scrotonin, and many other substances critical to health and well being. They are intimately involved in metabolism and glandular activity. Their presence is mandatory for glandular activity.

Amino acids are necessary for growth and cellular replication throughout the body. They are a major constituent for muscle, blood, skin, and internal organs. The proper functioning of the immune system is dependent on the presence of specific amino acids. They control the pathway that allows hormones and enzymes to be released. In addition to being the building blocks of structure, amino acids in effect turn on and off the 'chemical switches' that control our metabolism and body function.

Amino acids are involved in everything from our sense of thirst to how our brain functions. Messages from the brain that are sent to various body parts by neurological chemicals called neurotransmitters. These neurotransmitters are responsible for the complex messages and instructions that the brain sends to all body parts. Our feelings of alertness, anger, anxiety, thirst, hunger and all most sensations and feelings are controlled by organic chemicals, microtransmitters and glandular secretions or hormones.

The following amino acids and nutrients have an extremely positive effect on the anterior pituitary glands secretions of HGH.

a) L-arginine
b) L-ornithine
c) L-lysine and arginine pyroglutamate
d) OKG
e) L-glutamine/glutamine peptides
f) Glycine
g) Niacin/B_3
h) Vit. C
i) GABA

L-arginine: L-arginine is an essential amino acid. Arginine appears to increase the HGH levels by blocking the secretions of growth hormone inhibitor somatostatin. It is most effective used in a stack. It has been used by millions of athletes over the past 20 years to enhance production of HGH. It works even into old age, with one European study showing that it boosted blood levels of HGH to three times the level seen in their age group. The effects of arginine supplementation include increased fat burning and muscle building, enhanced immunity, and improving erectile function in men. It appears to work by blocking the hormone, somatostatin, which acts as a brake within the pituitary gland lowering the production and release of HGH. The most common dosage is four to 10 grams taken on an empty stomach one hour before exercise and before sleeping. Arginine also acts as a vasodilator.

L-ornithine: L-ornithine is a non-essential amino acid. It can be fabricated from arginine and is very similar in structure. It is also widely used to boost HGH. It has double the effectiveness of arginine at the same dosage. The usual dosage is two/three grams.

Arginine pyroglutamate: Arginine pyroglutamate must be used with L-lysine to achieve optimum results. It can be used with L-ornithine.

L-Lysine: It is an essential acid greatly increases the effect of arginine pyroglutamate when used together. Do not continue L-lysine with L-arginine. Lysine has a synergistic effect while arginine is pyroglutamine.

According to a 1981 study by Italian researcher, A. Isidori, M.D., and his associates at the University of Rome, the combination of 1,200 mg of lysine and 1,200 mg of arginine pyroglutamate, in 15 male volunteers, was 10 times more effective than taking arginine pyroglutamate alone. But another study by the Gerontology Research Centre in Baltimore found that L-lysine/L-arginine combination, even at twice the dosage, used in the Italian study failed to raise HGH levels. L-arginine and L-lysine compete for the same receptors. Arginine pyroglutamate attaches to a different receptor allowing for synergistic effect.

L-glutamine: L-glutamine is also known as conditional amino acid, meaning that there are reported conditions in which the body is unable to synthesise from other amino acids. It is the most abundant amino acids in the body. L-Glutamine is particularly valuable to the body during times of stress. The immune system is said to all but live on glutamine. Most effective used in a stack. The usual dosage is 3-8 grams.

Glutamine is the most recent amino acid to generate excitement as a HGH releaser. Tomas C Welbourne of Louisiana State University College of Medicine in Shreveport, in a 1995 study showed that a surprising small oral dose (about 2 grams of glutamine) raised HGH levels more than four times than when the subjects were given a placebo. Even more exciting, age did not diminish the response, at least in this small study of volunteers, who ranged from 32 to 64 years. The usual dose is 2-10 grams at bedtime and pre-exercise.

OKG: OKG is a French designer nutrient consisting of L-ornithine boundary to other molecules. It is a precursor to L-glutamine. In France it is used in hospitals to rebuild body tissue after surgery or trauma. The usual dosage is three/ten grams.

GABA: GABA is a non-essential amino acid. This, along with glutamine, is the most effective HGH secretagogue. GBB is synthesised from GABA and GBB is illegal because of recreational abuse. It improves REM sleep. More than two grams can produce extreme, but harmless, side effects. Usual dosage is three/five grams at night.

Niacin: B_3 using niacin in your amino acid stack results in a 30-40 per cent increase in HGH release. It can cause a harmless but initially scary flushing. It is a vasodilator. Take 250-500 mg with each amino stack.

DIETARY RECOMMENDATIONS

The American Heart Association (AHA), a leading authority on nutrition for more than 30 years, offers recommendations for healthy persons that apply whether you are active or not. The recommendations of AHA, those related to diet are given below:

a) Total fat intake should be no more than 30 per cent of calories.

b) Saturated fatty acid intake should be less than 10 per cent of calories. Saturated fatty acids are found primarily in animal fats, but also in palm, palm kernel and coconut oil.

c) Polyunsaturated fatty acid intake should be up to 10 per cent of calories. Corn, soybean and sunflower oil are examples of polyunsaturated fatty acids.

d) Monounsaturated fatty acids make up the rest of the total fat intake, about 10 to 15 per cent of total calories. Canola and olive oil are examples of monounsaturated oils.

e) Cholesterol intake should be less than 300 milligrams per day. It is found in foods from animals: beef, pork, mutton, poultry, fish, dairy products, egg yolks.

f) Limit sodium intake to no more than 2400 mg a day. To cut down on salt, use herbs and spices.

The following tips may help you to make an active person.

a) Eat a well-balanced diet that includes all kinds of foods.

b) Adjust your calorie intake to keep your ideal weight. Physical activity is the key to helping you achieve this goal.

c) Eat a diet fairly high in carbohydrates. Increase the amount of fruits, vegetables and other carbohydrates that you eat.

d) Drink fluids before, during and after a workout that lasts 30 minutes or more, especially in warm weather. While working out vigorously for 30-60 minutes or longer, drink six/eight ounces of fluid every 10-15 minutes.

e) Avoid salt tablets. Too much salt puts an extra burden on the kidneys. You can replace sodium lost during exercise with the food you eat.

f) Keep a daily weight chart in the hot summer months to check for hydration.

g) Avoid eating lots of sugar before you exercise. It may cause dehydration, stomach discomfort and low blood sugar.

h) Eating large portions of high-fat foods can delay digestion. So before you work out, eat carbohydrates such as bread, cereals and pasta. They are high-energy foods.

The US Recommended Daily Allowances are based on the RDA. The USRDA are listed below.

Food	*Functions*	*Recommendation*
Water	Maintains ability to deliver energy and oxygen to working muscles; maintains body temperature	6-8 glasses/day
Carbohydrates	Provides energy to body	50-55 per cent of total calories
Protein	Builds, repairs and maintains body tissues	15 per cent of total calories
Vitamins	Help regulate the body's chemical reactions	100 per cent of USRDA
Minerals	Form structures of the body and regulate body processes	100 per cent of USRDA
Electrolytes	Help maintain fluid	Sodium—no more than balance 2,400 mg per day; potassium—eat lots of fruits and vegetables
Fat	Provides a long-term source of energy	No more than 30 per cent of total calories

A suggested serving size of meat is about the size of a deck of cards. Some suggested serving sizes by weight include the following:

a) three ounces chicken, turkey, etc.

b) three ounces fish: flounder, cod, salmon, tuna, scallops

c) three ounces lean meat: beef, lamb, pork

d) two tablespoons peanut butter

e) one cup legumes.

Limit your egg consumption to three/four egg yolks or less per week, including those used in cooking.

Five or more servings daily. A suggested serving size is:

Vegetables	*Fruit*
1/2 to 1 cup cooked or raw	1/2 cup juice or 1 medium-size piece

a) *One serving should be a good source of vitamin C*: asparagus, broccoli, cabbage, tomatoes, berries, cantaloupe, orange, papaya, strawberries, tangerines, etc.

b) *One serving should be a good source of vitamin A*: broccoli, carrots, sweet potatoes, leafy greens, kale, peas, rutabagas, spinach, string beans, watercress, winter squash, yellow corn.

Six or more servings daily. A suggested serving size is:

a) one slice whole-grain breads

b) one/three cup cooked cereal

c) one cup flaked cereal

d) one cup pasta or rice

e) three cups popcorn (no fat added)

f) six salt crackers

Adults—two/three servings; children and adolescents—three/four servings daily. A suggested serving size is:

a) one cup skim milk, one/two per cent or one per cent

b) one cup non-fat or low-fat yogurt

c) one/two to one cup low fat cottage cheese

d) one ounce low-fat cheese (made with low-fat or skim milk)

e) one/two cup ice milk.

Restrict fats if necessary for weight control. A suggested serving size is:

a) one teaspoon oil—safflower, corn, sunflower, soybean, olive, canola

b) one teaspoon margarine

c) two teaspoons no-fat or low-fat mayonnaise

d) two teaspoons no-fat or low-fat mayonnaise-type salad dressing

e) two teaspoons sunflower or pumpkin seeds

f) one tablespoon nuts.

If you are watching your weight, use these items moderately—one to two servings daily. Choose low-calorie, low-fat desserts and sweets such as fresh fruit, sherbet, ices or any dessert made from ingredients listed in the food plan.

If you train an hour or more a day, plan high-carbohydrate, high-protein snacks to meet your energy needs. Low-fat fruit yogurt or a whole-wheat sandwich with an ounce of lean turkey and a piece of fruit are two examples of good snacks. A cup of dry cereal mixed with raisins or other dry fruit can be packed in plastic bags for snacks away from home.

Athletes can also add juice and sports drinks that have glucose polymers to meet their fluid, carbohydrate and electrolyte needs. Contact a local registered dietitian or licensed nutritionist in your area if you need help planning snacks or guidance in fluid/ electrolyte drinks.

Liberal amounts of carbohydrates—bread, pasta, potatoes, cereal—help you keep high levels of muscle and liver glycogen. This is how athletes improve their endurance. There are many ways to load up on them. Most increase the carbohydrate content of the diet to 65 per cent or more for three days before a race or critical training session. You should reduce your training during this time and rest your muscles to allow them to become saturated with carbohydrates.

Do not use this method more than a few times a year. And use it only for events that last one/two hours or longer.

A carbohydrate-loading programme may lead to several harmful side effects. For example, increased fluid could result in swollen joints. If you are a young adult and at risk for heart disease or other chronic disorders, avoid this programme.

On the day before your event, choose fibre-rich carbohydrates such as:

a) wheat bread;
b) bran cereal;
c) bran muffins;
d) fruits; and
e) vegetables.

Eat your largest meal at noon. That way, your food will have plenty of time to digest and pass through your system. Also, drink extra fluid to hydrate your system. On the morning of the event eat a light breakfast. Eating sugar before activities that last less than 20-30 minutes offers little physiological benefit. The reason is that the energy stored as glycogen in your liver and muscles is sufficient to maintain your blood sugar levels. You can control your weight by keeping a balance between the calories you eat and burn. All unused calories are stored as body fat. Some body fat insulates and protects vital organs. But too much body fat will make it harder for you to move around and enjoy physical activity.

Use body fat percentages as a general guide for achieving a high fitness level. Desirable percentages of body fat are about 20-25 per cent for women and 10-15 per cent for men. Some highly trained athletes may have much lower body fat. Older athletes may have slightly higher body fat levels than younger athletes. But they usually don't train as hard or as much. Many fitness clubs have staff who measure body fat percentages. If you don't belong to a club, a licensed nutritionist, registered dietitian or qualified health professional can help you. To reduce the amount of excess fat on your body, reduce your fat intake and increase your physical activity. Regular exercise is the key to maintain your ideal weight. In fact, it:

a) improves appetite control;
b) minimises loss of muscle tissue;
c) 'burns' calories and cuts body fat; and
d) promotes a feeling of well-being.

If you like moving your body, you will always be young enough to exercise. But follow proper guidelines to help reduce your risk of injury. No two bodies are the same. So make sure your programme fits your needs. Most people do not need to see a doctor before they start a gradual, sensible exercise programme. But see a doctor first if you are older than 40; already at risk for heart disease; or haven't exercised in recent years. Your doctor can give you tests that can help determine how long, hard and often you can work out. To condition your heart and lungs, you must bring your heart rate to a certain point, called thc targct heart rate zone.

When you stop exercising, quickly place the tips of your first two fingers lightly over one of the carotid arteries on your neck. These blood vessels are located to the left or right of your Adam's apple. Count your pulse for 10 seconds and multiply by six. Your target heart rate depends on your age and maximum heart rate. Usually your maximum heart rate is determined by subtracting your age from 220. Your target heart rate is 50-75 per cent of your maximum heart rate, depending on how far you have advanced in your exercise programme. After six months of regular exercise, you can exercise at up to 85 per cent of your maximum heart rate.

HEALTH AT ANY SIZE

There was a time when the fat, voluptuous woman was considered a thing of beauty. But today, we think of fat people as objects of ridicule. To be fat in America is to be considered a modern-day pariah. Fashion, magazines, and movies continually reinforce the notion that only thin is beautiful; only thin is acceptable. "We have confused thinness with health," says health writer Laura Fraser. "We've sort of mixed our beauty ideals with our medical ideals, and we think they're the same when in fact they're not." Fraser, who has written extensively on health issues, says there is growing evidence that being overweight is not as big a health risk as we used to think.

The Cooper Institute For Aerobics Research in Dallas found that the biggest factor in determining how long someone lives is not how much they weigh, but how much they exercise. Their study showed that men who were thin but unfit had three times the rate of early death as men who were fat but fit. "Aside from people on the extremes, a lot of studies show that what really counts is how much you exercise," adds Fraser.

Obesity-related conditions are the second leading cause of preventable death, putting people at increased risk of high blood pressure, diabetes, heart disease. The medical community has been sitting on the sidelines while the disease of obesity has mushroomed into a public health crisis. Yet, the long-standing gospel about fat is changing. Scientists say a more relevant health indicator is body shape. For instance. people shaped like pears—carrying much of their weight on the hips and thighs—are much less likely to have cardiovascular problems than those shaped like apples—where fat is carried above the waist.

According to Joanne Ikeda, a nutrition educator at UC Berkeley, our weight is simply a poor indicator of how healthy we are. She says: "It really plays a very small and, perhaps, insignificant role. The much more important thing is that people maintain a healthy lifestyle because that is what is going to reduce their risk of disease."

Some people simply do not believe you can be healthy at any size. But in defiance of those beliefs, a growing number of women say they are proving that they are fat and fit. Virtually all experts agree that exercise is vital to good health.

ULTIMATE AEROBIC EXERCISE AND FITNESS PROGRAMME

The Ultimate Aerobic and Anaerobic Exercise Programme provides an environment for an injury-free aerobic and anaerobic workout. This multi-faceted exercise/workout programme systematically exercises all the major muscle groups of the body in a thorough aerobic and resistive fashion.

There are almost as many claimed benefits of exercise or fitness programme as there are aerobic exercise videos. Some of these benefits are physiological, some psychological, some a combination of the two, and some fantasy and some illogical, magical unbelievable TV marketing hype.

Current research supports a complete fitness programme which include:

a) anaerobic exercise, optimised with circuit training;
b) aerobic exercise, optimised with interval training; and
c) some stretching or yoga.

For hormonal stimulation and weight loss do the aerobics first. This will deplete blood glucose and stimulate fat metabolism for energy. You will tend to 'bonk' or run out of energy during the anaerobic portion of the programme. The lower your blood glucose is when you exercise the more of a HGH spike you will get because HGH is part of the fat metabolism equation. For optimal muscle gains you can do the anaerobic before the aerobic, this will allow for plenty of blood glucose energy for the weight lifting anaerobic portion of your programme.

The consensus is that the level of exercise for hormonal stimulation must be somewhat harder than the level of exercise required for cardiovascular benefit. There are increases in HGH associated with relatively hard aerobics and relatively heavy anaerobic exercise.

Participants in the Ultimate Aerobic and Anaerobic Synergistic Exercise Programme will experience increased serum levels of HGH. HGH peaks when blood glucose is low, the best time for HGH stimulating exercise in the morning after the all night fast and 30 minutes after the HGH stimulating amino acid secretagogue stack. If you cannot exercise first thing in the morning, time your meals so that you have several hours (two/three or more) to burn off the blood glucose from the meal before you workout.

Do anaerobics, heavier muscle building weightlifting, after the aerobic portion of your workout. The aerobics will deplete blood glucose which will result in even higher HGH levels. A relatively hard, planned and synergistic workout will result in up to a 250 per cent increase in HGH secretion. Low blood sugar/glucose is conducive to HGH increases but are also conducive to 'bonking' (running out of energy).

REFERENCES

Berg, F., 'Nondiet movement gains strength', *Obesity and Health* 6:85-90, 1992.

Foreyt, J.P. and G. K. Goodrick, 'Weight management without dieting', *Nutrition Today* 28 (2): 4-9, 1993.

Occupational Health Nursing Care Guidelines, Daly-Gawenda, Debra, Hudson, Edsel K., Perea, Carol (eds.) Paperback ISBN: 0826193501.

Oil That Heals: A Physicians Successes With Caster Oil Treatments, Mcgarey, William A., Paperback ISBN: 0876043082.

Oil-Protein Diet Cookbook, Budwig, Johanna, Paperback, ISBN: 0969527225.

Omega 3 Oils, Rudin, Donald Paperback ISBN: 0895297213.

Omega Diet, Wills, Judith Paperback ISBN: 074727195X.

Omega Diet: The Lifesaving Nutritional Program Based On The Diet Of The Island Of Crete, Simopoulos, Artemis P. Paperback, ISBN: 0060930233.

Omichinski, Linda and Kathleen Harrison,'Nondiet Weight Management: A Lifestyle Approach to Health and Fitness', San Marcos, *Nutrition Dimension,* 1995.

Scott K. Powers Stephen L. Dodd, *Total Fitness: Exercise, Nutrition, and Wellness*, 1999.

3

Healthy Eating

Food has been considered medicine for the body for centuries. Food is a staple of life, and the food you consume contributes to the length and quality of your life. The types of food you eat actually controls your health and how you look. Staying healthy means eating healthy, eating nutritiously. It is imperative to eat foods that are nutrient rich, foods that are high in vitamins and minerals. If you eat foods loaded with fat and sugar you will probably feel sluggish and be overweight. Balance and moderation in diet are keys to successful eating.

Food is fuel for the body and eating more nutritious food will keep your body going longer. We all want to live longer, feel better, look good and improve our longevity for which we need to be more fastidious with what and how much we eat every day. It may seem obvious, but eating right is one of the first steps in living a healthy life. If you are impatient to lose weight, you may leave your common sense at home while searching for quick, easy and potentially dangerous solutions. Take a look at your health habits for the past five years, along with your genetic heritage, and you may find the real answers to your weight problem. Five safe weight loss tips are:

a) Eat a balanced diet.

b) Remember the basics of weight loss.

c) You need to eat fewer calories than your body needs.

d) Reducing intake by 500 calories a day, will help you lose one pound a week.

e) Do not go below 1,200 calories a day; your diet quality will suffer and you will not lose any faster.

The key to healthy eating is the time-testing advice of balance, variety and moderation. Eat a wide variety of foods without getting too many calories or too much of any one nutrient. The following guidelines can help you follow that advice while still enjoying the foods you eat.

a) *Eat a variety of nutrient-rich foods*: You need more than 40 different nutrients for good health, and no single food supplies them all. Your daily food selection should include bread and other wholegrain products; fruits; vegetables; dairy products; and meat, poultry, fish and other protein foods. How much you should eat depends on your calorie needs.
b) *Enjoy plenty of wholegrains, fruits and vegetables*: Surveys show most people eat enough of these foods. Do you eat 6-11 servings from the bread, rice, cereal and pasta group, three of which should be wholegrains? Do you eat 24 servings of fruit and three-five servings of vegetables? If you do not enjoy some of these at first, give them another chance. Look through cookbooks for tasty ways to prepare unfamiliar foods.
c) *Maintain a healthy weight*: The weight that is right for you depends on many factors including your sex, height, age and heredity. Excess body fat increases your chances for high blood pressure, heart disease, stroke, diabetes, some types of cancer and other illnesses. But being too thin can increase your risk for osteoporosis, menstrual irregularities and other health problems. If you're constantly losing and regaining weight, a registered dietitian can help you develop sensible eating habits for successful weight management. Regular exercise is also important to maintaining a healthy weight.

d) *Eat moderate portions*: If you keep portion sizes reasonable, it is easier to eat the foods you want and stay healthy. Did you know the recommended serving of cooked meat is three ounces, similar in size to a deck of playing cards? A medium piece of fruit is one serving and a cup of pasta equals two servings. A pint of ice-cream contains four servings.

e) *Eat regular meals*: Skipping meals can lead to out-of-control hunger, often resulting in overeating. When you are very hungry, it is also tempting to forget about good nutrition. Snacking between meals can help curb hunger, but don't eat so much that your snack becomes an entire meal.

f) *Reduce, do not eliminate certain foods*: Most people eat for pleasure as well as nutrition. If your favourite foods are high in fat, salt or sugar, the key is moderating how much of these foods you eat and how often you eat them.

   Identify major sources of these ingredients in your diet and make changes, if necessary. Adults who eat high-fat meats or whole-milk dairy products at every meal are probably eating too much fat. Use the nutrition facts panel on the food label to help balance your choices.

   Choosing skim or low-fat dairy products and lean cuts of meat such as flank steak and beef round can reduce fat intake significantly.

   If you love fried chicken, however, you don't have to give it up. Just eat it less often. When dining out, share it with a friend, ask for a take-home bag or a smaller portion.

g) *Balance your food choices over-time*: Not every food has to be perfect. When eating a food high in fat, salt or sugar, select other foods that are low in these ingredients. If you miss out on any food group one day, make up for it the next. Your food choices over several days should fit together into a healthy pattern.

h) *Know your diet pitfalls*: To improve your eating habits, you first have to know what is wrong with them. Write down everything you eat for three days. Then check your list according to the rest of these tips. Do you add a lot of butter, creamy sauces or salad dressings? Rather than eliminating these foods, just cut back your portions. Are you getting enough fruits and vegetables? If not, you may be missing out on vital nutrients.

i) *Make changes gradually*: Just as there are no super-foods or easy answers to a healthy diet, don't expect to totally revamp your eating habits overnight. Changing too much, too fast can get in the way of success. Begin to remedy excesses or deficiencies with modest changes that can add up to positive, lifelong eating habits. For instance, if you are not liking the taste of skim milk, try low-fat. Eventually you may find you like skim, too.

j) *Remember, foods are not good or bad*: Select foods based on your total eating patterns, not whether any individual food is good or bad. Do not feel guilty if you love foods such as apple pie, potato chips, candy bars or ice-cream. Eat them in moderation, and choose other foods to provide the balance and variety that are vital to good health.

ROLE OF FAT IN FITNESS

With so much information available about the effects of dietary fat on health, understanding the role fat plays in a well-balanced diet can be pretty confusing. To cut through the confusion, it is important to remember that fat is an essential nutrient that everyone needs to stay healthy. Fat is a valuable energy source and carries fat-soluble vitamins needed for proper growth and development. It also contributes important taste and textural qualities. However, too much fat will increase the risk of heart disease, obesity and other health problems.

All fats are a combination of saturated, polyunsaturated and monounsaturated fatty acids. Each of these types of fats have different effects on the body, but all contain nine calories per gram. Blood cholesterol levels are influenced by family history, weight, age, smoking, physical activity and eating habits. Studies have shown that diets which are too high in certain saturated fatty acids and dietary cholesterol can raise the blood cholesterol.

Although fat does have double the calories of carbohydrates and proteins, essential fats do give you a major advantage in getting lean. Too many times we have been told that all fats are bad. That fat makes you fat. This has made many of us scared of all fats and has helped to promote the no-fat or low-fat craze. Go to any grocery store and you will see aisle after aisle of fat-free foods. This would seem to presume that all fats are the same. While many fats are not good, especially those that are hydrogenated, fried or heat processed, it is very important to know that not all fats are created equally. Some fats are essential because your body cannot make them on its own. It is these essential fats that also help you burn body fat.

One of the main reasons essentials fats help improve your metabolism is they balance your body's ratio of insulin to glucagon. When you eat sugary foods, the hormone insulin is secreted to remove the excess sugar from your body. But when too much insulin is released due to excessively sugary meals, i.e., refined and processed bread, pastas, tropical fruits, it blocks the critical pancreatic hormone glucagon from operating effectively within your body. Essential fats help balance the insulin levels, so that glucagon can be better released to unlock the body's fat storage banks and begin converting unwanted body-fat into energy.

Furthermore, eating essential fats increases your metabolism by helping to activate a very special type of fat that lies deep into your body surrounding vital organs such as the heart, kidneys and adrenal glands. It also cushions the spinal column as well as the neck and major thoracic blood vessels. The body-fat we want to burn, which lies near the top of our skin, is technically called white fat.

The brown fat is completely unique because it burns calories for heat rather than retaining those calories for future use. Brown fat is not a storage fat like white fat but rather a calorie-burning engine. Although brown fat makes up 10 per cent or less of total body fat, it is responsible for 25 per cent of all the fat calories burned by all the other body tissues.

The best essential fats you can eat are the omega fats. Three of the most well known and well-researched omega fats are the omega-3s, omega-6s and the omega-9s. Right now a very simple thing you can do to start benefiting from these fat-burning oils is to start using extra-virgin olive oil in place of butter.

ROLE OF PROTEIN IN FITNESS

Since we are going to be focused on building your lean muscle tissue you will need to make sure you are eating the right amounts of protein. Protein is the body's building material. The reason you need to eat protein is to provide your body with the materials it needs to build, repair and maintain your lean muscle tissue. Furthermore, over half of your dry body weight is made from protein. This not only includes muscle tissue but hair, skin, nails, blood, hormones, enzymes, brain cells and much more.

Without enough protein you actually start to break down and recycle existing body, protein to supply your body with the amino acids that your food intake is lacking. When this protein breakdown occurs it is the worst thing that can happen because you sacrifice muscle and your metabolism slows down. As a result, your body actually burns less body-fat.

ROLE OF CARBOHYDRATES IN FITNESS

Carbohydrates are important energy sources, fuelling the central nervous system and muscles during physical activity. Supplying four calories per gram, carbohydrates also help the body efficiently use vitamins, minerals, amino acids and other essential nutrients. Scientists classify carbohydrates into two categories: simple and complex.

Sugars are called simple carbohydrates because they consist of one or two sugars units. Sugars occur naturally in fruits, vegetables, milk and other foods, as well as in a refined state, such as table sugar or sucrose. The body cannot distinguish between naturally-occurring and added sugars and digests both in exactly the same manner.

Complex carbohydrates, found in grain foods, fruits and vegetables, get their name from their complex chain-like structure of many sugar units. Included in this category are starches and dietary fibre. During digestion, starch is typically broken down into sugars and used by the body for energy.

High-fibre diets can reduce the risks of heart disease and certain types of cancer. Soluble fibre in cereals, oatmeal, beans and other foods has been found to lower blood cholesterol. Insoluble fibre in cauliflower, cabbage and other vegetables and fruits helps move foods through the stomach and intestine, thereby decreasing the risk of cancers of the colon and rectum. Wholegrain breads and cereals, dry beans and peas, fruits and vegetables are generally low in fat, contain little or no cholesterol and are rich in fibre, which facilitates proper bowel function and can reduce symptoms of chronic constipation, diverticular disease and haemorrhoids.

The Association of Official Analytic Chemists International (AOACI) has stated that complex carbohydrates can be described as the sum of available starches and fibre, including resistant starch and oligosaccharides and lignin. Based on this definition, AOACI also believes analytical methods can be developed to measure complex carbohydrates. However, until such methods are developed and complex carbohydrate information is included on the food label, many nutritionists say it will be difficult to improve consumers' consumption of complex carbohydrates.

The quick checklist given below will help you to determine whether you are consuming the recommended three servings of wholegrain foods per day. Look for the words 'wholegrain' near the beginning of the ingredient list on the food-label.

Wholegrain foods

a) One serving

Wholegrain cereals

a) one cup dry

b) one/two cup cooked

Wholegrain breads

a) one/two bagel

b) one slice bread

c) one small roll

Wholegrain pasta

a) one/two cup cooked or brown rice

b) foods made with wholegrain flour

c) two small pancakes

d) one small waffle

e) thre/four crackers.

DIETING AND FITNESS

Weight loss is simple, just eat less. If you starve off unwanted weight you will not win. By just eating less or drinking diet type shakes or just eating meal replacement bars, research shows that up to 50 per cent of the weight loss comes from muscle tissue loss, not fat loss. When you don't eat enough the thyroid gland tries to protect you from starvation. What it does is it secretes less thyroxine. Thyroxine is a hormone that helps to regulate your metabolism and the less thyroxine secreted the slower the metabolism and the fewer calories you burn. And if you continue on a stringent diet for a long period of time what happens is your body will eventually start to consume itself. You might think this is what you want because it will get you to lose weight.

Unless you continue not eating, once you start eat normally your body will regain the weight lost. You might think that you would be no worse off than when you started. Since you also lost lean tissue it gets even harder to lose the same weight again. The weight you regain will be 100 per cent fat and there will be more. Remember that the goal is to burn fat and never lose muscle tissue.

You will also need to eat carbohydrates, because they play a critical part in achieving fat loss. Yes, you heard right, carbohydrates can be used to get you lean. Avoid simple carbohydrates that are high on the glycemic index and eat complex carbohydrates that are much lower in the glycemic index. Simple carbohydrates are foods that are refined and processed such as white rice, white flour, white pasta and white sugar.

Complex carbohydrates are foods that are usually wholegrain and unprocessed. Complex carbohydrates provide you just the right amount of time-released energy that, when released in a regulated manner, act as a lighter fluid or kindling that helps you burn excess body-fat.

By trickling in small amounts of complex carbohydrates, the fat will burn long and steady. Dump too much lighter fluid at one time and you get a flash fire that flares quickly and then burns out almost immediately. Unlike simple carbohydrates, complex carbohydrates do not rapidly release into your bloodstream because of their complex molecular structure. This means that complex carbohydrates never overwhelm your body with sugar rushes because they take more time to break down. Thus they provide the ideal amounts of time-released sugar to burn fat. This allows your body to use body-fat as its primary fuel. So the key is eating complex, not simple carbohydrates. If you want to eat bread, pasta or bagels they must be ones that are made from ingredients containing complex carbohydrates.

Although vegetables are a type of carbohydrate, they are grouped in their own category because of their unique beneficial effects on fat loss. Vegetables are very high in water content, which means that they are also very high in oxygen. In order for our lean muscle tissue to burn fat it needs oxygen to help convert the fat into energy. When you eat vegetables you will be flooding your body with water which will dramatically increase your oxygen levels, thus improving your metabolism.

Vegetables are high in fibre, and ounce for ounce, are probably the most filling low-calorie food you can eat. Since vegetables need to be chewed more and take longer to consume this gives your brain time to realise that you are eating and turns off the hunger switch sooner. Most vegetables are also very low in simple sugars. They also have almost no calories. New research has shown that green vegetables contain elements called phytochemicals that form a plant's immune system. These phytochemicals also act to keep the human immune system strong.

DIET ESSENTIALS

Dietary Fibres

Dietary fibre generally refers to those parts of fruits, vegetables, grains, nuts and legumes that can't be digested by humans. Meats and dairy products do not contain fibre. There are two basic types of fibre—insoluble and soluble. Most fibres containing foods feature both, but one or the other type often predominates in specific parts of a food and determines the characteristic texture of that portion of the food.

Insoluble fibres produce the tough, chewy feel of wheat kernels, popcorn, apple skin and nuts. Essential to the cellular structure of plants, insoluble fibres include cellulose, hemicelluloses and lignin. They do not dissolve in water.

Soluble fibres include pectin, gums, mucilages and algal polysaccharides. Although pectin is part of cell walls, most soluble fibres are found within plant cells. The gummy essence of oat bran and the musky centre of a cooked kidney bean reflect both the soluble fibre content of those foods and the ability of soluble fibres to soak up water.

The fibre content of a food varies according to the species of the plant and stage of maturation, but seeds, berries, fruit skins and the bran layers of cereal grains generally contain larger amounts of a plant's fibre. A diet that is high in fibre is found to be protective against colon cancer and possible cardiovascular diseases. A high-fibre diet appears to reduce disease risk by increasing faecal bulk decreasing the transit time of food through the gastrointestinal tract, reducing blood cholesterol levels and helping to control blood sugar levels.

With their distinct physical characteristics, insoluble and soluble fibres work differently. Insoluble fibres seem to have their greatest impact on the health of the colon or large intestine. Large amounts of insoluble fibres increase faecal bulk and draw water into the large intestine. The result is a larger, softer stool that exerts less pressure on the colon walls and is eliminated more quickly. Indeed, the most well-established benefit of a high-fibre diet is in the treatment and prevention of constipation. The reduced pressure also may help prevent diverticulosis.

Large amounts of insoluble fibres dilute the concentration of potential carcinogens that may be present in the stool, and the decreased transit time reduces the exposure of the intestinal wall to those substances. Furthermore, insoluble fibres alter the pH of the large intestine, interfering with microbial activity that produces carcinogens. The combined effect may be a reduced risk of colon cancer. Complementing the action of insoluble fibres, some soluble fibres also add to faecal bulk and increase its water content. But the soluble fibre's potential for reducing blood cholesterol levels recently has grabbed the spotlight.

Diets rich in soluble fibres such as oat bran may help reduce total cholesterol and low density lipoprotein (LDL) cholesterol in people with both high and normal blood cholesterol levels. A diet low in fat and high in soluble fibre may reduce an individual's blood cholesterol by three per cent to six per cent.

Soluble fibres appear to reduce blood cholesterol in two ways. First, they prevent the re-absorption of vital bile acids from the small intestine. To replace the lost bile acids, cholesterol is drawn from the body, thereby reducing its cholesterol supply. Second, the fermentation of soluble fibres in the intestine produces short-chain fatty acids which block the synthesis of cholesterol.

Table 2.1. Sources of fibre

Insoluble fibre	*Soluble fibre*	*Soluble / insoluble fibres*
wheat bran	oat bran	citrus fruits
whole wheat products	whole grain oats	psyllium
corn bran	barley	pectin
brown rice	navy beans	carrageenan
rice bran	soyabean	guar gum
bananas	kidney beans	flax seed
cauliflower	apples	
nuts	potatoes	
lentils	broccoli	
green beans	carrots	
green peas		

Soluble fibres also may help control the rise in blood sugar following a meal and reduce insulin requirements in some patients with diabetes mellitus. By increasing the viscosity of gastrointestinal contents, soluble fibres retard gastric emptying, slowing the absorption of glucose in the process.

Food composition databases today reflect the crude fibre content of food, which is determined by subjecting food to a chemical treatment that destroys large amounts of its insoluble fibres and almost all of its soluble fibres. The resulting value seriously underestimates the true dietary fibre content of food, which has been judged to be three to five times higher. This created difficulties when attempting to evaluate fibre intake.

Methods that provide a more accurate reading are now in limited use. The neutral detergent fibre method is primarily useful in estimating insoluble fibre content. The total dietary fibre (TDF) method is the only process that estimates total fibre content. Modification of the TDF method also allows determination of soluble and insoluble fractions, but provisional databases using figures derived from this method currently do not reflect the type of fibre in a food.

The diet and health report of the US National Academy of Sciences advises a daily intake of five or more servings of fruits and vegetables and six or more servings of wholegrain breads and cereals and legumes. Health professionals caution against making an immediate leap from a low-fibre intake to recommended levels. Increasing fibre consumption too rapidly can result in flatulence, cramping and intestinal distention. Undesirable side effects may be avoided through the gradual addition of fibre to the diet along with an adequate fluid intake.

People consuming well-balanced and varied diets high in fibre are unlikely to experience mineral deficiencies. While fibre does seem significant to human health, scientists stress its interplay with other factors must not be ignored. The effects of heredity, the quality of the overall diet and habits such as smoking and exercise can outweigh any single dietary modification.

Importance of Sodium

Sodium is one of two principal determinants of blood volume or extracellular fluid in the body. The other determinant is plasma and protein count, which changes over a much longer period of time. Blood volume is regulated precisely by the kidneys over 24 hours, such that all sodium chloride ingested the previous day is excreted in the urine—except for losses due to sweating, lactation or hemorrhaging. The kidneys know exactly how much excess sodium must be eliminated from the body to maintain proper blood volume, which is essential for life.

Blood pressure is the product of total blood volume times its resistance inside the human circulatory system or vascular tree. If system resistance is relatively low, the same blood volume will result in lower blood pressure. Conversely, the same blood volume facing high resistance would result in high blood pressure. About 95 per cent of the sodium salts in our diets are sodium chloride or table salt; the remainder are derived from sodium bicarbonate, mineral water, etc.

Dietary sodium restriction has a heterogeneous effect on blood pressure. That is, for some people sodium restriction causes a decrease in blood pressure, for some it has no effect on the blood pressure and for others it actually causes a clinically significant increase in blood pressure.

Since the 1980s, there have been a number of studies suggesting that potassium, calcium, magnesium and other minerals can influence blood pressure response to dietary sodium. Studies suggest that restricting sodium chloride can lower blood pressure, provided these other electrolytes are also present in the diet in sufficient amounts. Those with sufficient intakes of these minerals appear to be able to consume the highest levels of sodium with minimal impact on blood pressure.

Older people are at greater risk of developing hypertension because of their decreased efficiency in absorbing minerals through the gut and their decreased renal efficiency in maintaining electrolyte balance. But not all elderly need to restrict their sodium intake; in fact, some can develop dizziness and hypotension if they do not maintain adequate sodium chloride intake.

FOODS TO EAT AND AVOID

The food stuffs to be taken or avoid, amonut of intake, reasons for take or avoid, are briefly described below.

Foods to Eat

Foodstuff	*Amount*	*Why it is essential*
Vegetables	Any amount; dark coloured ones are best. Fresh and little processed is preferred.	The coloured ones have many types of carotenoids and flavonoids that prevent cancer, heart and vascular troubles, strokes, etc.
Grains and rice	Any amount: if tolerated	Basic food; contains many good components like fibre, mineral and vitamins that are removed in refining.
Beans, soy and legumes	Reasonable amounts; combines with grains	Lower bad cholesterol and triglycerides. High fibre, low fat. Combine with nuts and grains. Their protein may be good for the heart. Soy is good for health, heart and anti-cancer but there's discussion if its extracted protein and hormone-like ingredients are healthy.

Contd...

Foodstuff	*Amount*	*Why it is essential*
Fibre	About 30 g/day. This is average intake. 50g/day really helps diabetes control.	Often missing processed foods. Aids elimination — reducing colon cancer risk by about 1/3rd. Each gram/ day lowers LDL cholesterol by nearly one per cent. Found in whole grains, fruits, beans, vegetables. 2 tablespoons of crushed flax seed gets you most of your fibre and all your omega-3; it also lowers bad and Lp (a) cholesterol and helps keep you regular.
Fruits and berries	Lots, within reason	Lots of vitamins and fibre and no fats. Their flavonoids strengthen blood vessels and are strong antioxidants.
Eggs	Regularly	High in protein, B-vitamins, lecthin and choline. High in cholesterol but low in fat. Normally proportionally raise good cholesterol more than bad. Avoid anything with dried egg-powder or dried liver.
Meats	Not essential. Some factory animal farming is ecologically, morally and nutritionally good.	As fresh as possible. Aging and over-frying damages or oxidises fats which make the basically good LDL go bad and are best avoided.

Contd...

Foodstuff	*Amount*	*Why it is essential*
Oils	2 tablespoons of flax or fish oil, or 2 tbsp. canola or unhydrogenated soyabean oil	The only 2 essential oils (vitamin F) are linolenic (n-6 or omega-6) and alpha linolenic (n-3 or omega-3). These 2 polysaturates are the feed-stock for 3 classes of hormones and for nerve, brain, skin, and cell walls. Omega-3's vital role is compromised by heating and hydrogenation, by shortening, by omega-6s and by most saturated fats.
Alcohol	1-2 glasses of red-wine/day	Low amounts reduce heart disease. Red wine with its flavonoids protects blood cholesterol. Best with foods containing B vitamins such as liver. Alcohol + folic acid appear to be cardio protective while folic acid may well reduce the risk of some cancers linked to alcohol intake.
Lecithin	1-2 table spoons per day	Emulsifies fat; improves types of blood fats. It is a part of our nerves and brain; forms choline and betaine; Health food store granules have nice fatty flavour.
Water	Lots—within reason	Keeps things fluid and may cut bladder cancer by ½.

Contd...

Foods to Avoid

Foodstuff	*Amount*	*Why to avoid*
Solid fats from lands and animals	Limit these saturated fats, but some are needed	Zero fibre, vitamins or essential oils. They compete with the good oils for nutrients and do slowdown some essential cell functions, yet are part of others.
Trans and deep fried oils	Tasty but toxic, There is no nutritional excuse to hydrogenate anything and many reasons not to.	Man-made hardened oils. Made from and interfere with essential omega-3 and 6-oils. They lower good and raise bad cholesterol in nearly all store-bought baked goods made with shortening.
Oils of corn, sunflower or unrefined industrial types.	Avoid	High intake of refined omega-6 oils like corn, sunflower, safflower, linola and cotton generate too much of one class of hormones. This can cause irregular heart rhythm, cramps and other heart problems.
Flour (white refined) Most store-bought pasta.	Avoid The removed bran and germs are amazingly good sources of minerals and vitamins	They lack essential nutrients. They are linked to increased heart disease. Dried egg noodles have dangerous oxidised cholesterol.

Contd...

Foodstuff	*Amount*	*Why to avoid*
White rice	Avoid	Use the nutritionally superior and good-for-the-heart brown rice.
Sugar	Avoid	The fructose half-refined sugar is a building block for cholesterol.
Diary	Not essential for adults	Seventy-five per cent of world's population has some problems to digest cow's milk. Aged cheese has oxidised cholesterol.

EATING DISORDERS

Eating disorders receive considerable attention and are prevalent in today's society. Hundred years ago the first case of *anorexia nervosa*, or self-induced starvation, was documented in England. Yet, it stands to reason that even before the term anorexia was coined, many people struggling with eating disorders were simply diagnosed as having another ailment. Eating disorders threaten physical health, psychological well-being and sometimes life. Since many people with these problems suffer alone and do not seek professional help, it is difficult to determine the precise number of cases in the US.

The American Psychiatric Association (APA) estimates that at any given time, 500,000 people are battling eating disorders. The APA's 1993 *Practice Guidelines* estimate that between one and four per cent of adolescents and young adults are afflicted. Although the typical patient is a white, middle to upper middle class young woman, some researchers report an increasing number of cases among males and women of other age and ethnic groups.

The APA recognised two eating disorders: *anorexia nervosa* and *bulimia nervosa*. Cases of *anorexia nervosa* and *bulimia nervosa* have doubled over the past decade, according to the National Centre for Health Statistics (NCHS). Binge-eating, although not yet a recognised eating disorder, is receiving considerable attention as a related disorder. The major weight loss associated with *anorexia nervosa* results in a total body weight at least 15 per cent below the range of normal weight for age and height. Overtime, women suffering from this disorder stop menstruating and may damage vital organs including the heart and brain. Anorexia is believed to affect between one-half and one per cent of women in late adolescence and early adulthood, according to the APA.

Bulimia nervosa is a serious eating disorder typified by binging followed by either self-induced vomiting, use of laxatives, diuretics or enemas, strict dieting or fasting, or vigorous exercise in order to rid the body of the food and prevent weight gain. Although some victims of *anorexia nervosa* also exhibit symptoms of *bulimia nervosa*, it is recognised as a distinct disorder. *Bulimia nervosa* is believed to affect between one and three per cent of adolescents and young women in the US, although estimates among college-age women reach as high as one out of every five. *Bulimia nervosa* victims often are able to hide their problems because they eat normally in public and binge-and-purge in secret. Symptoms of *bulimia nervosa*, which may be obvious to family and friends, include a chronically inflamed and sore throat that may bleed, decaying tooth enamel and swollen salivary glands in the neck and jaw which can make the face appear puffy.

Binge-eating is another important type of eating disorder. Although less is known about binge-eating disorder, recent estimates suggest that as many as two per cent of the general population and 30 per cent of individuals attending hospital affiliated weight control programmes may be afflicted. Binge-eating, which has been proposed for official recognition as a diagnostic category of eating disorder, is similar to *bulimia nervosa* in that sufferers may consume extraordinary amounts of food during a single binge. However, they do not compensate for the binge by purging.

Most eating disorder specialists acknowledge that the disorders are very complex and likely to involve physical, psychological, societal, cultural and familial aspects. The development of an eating disorder is not triggered solely by the desire to be thin. Family dynamics often contribute to the development of an eating disorder. Some people with eating disorders come from enmeshed families where emotional, relational and physical space boundaries may be too blurry. This 'enmeshment' inhibits independence and the development of a separate self.

A prominent theory about eating disorders—that the person with the eating disorder is trying to gain some measure of control in her life—is consistent with this type of family structure. For some people, the act of dieting itself provides an illusion of control. Depression, feelings of inadequacy, anxiety and loneliness, stress and anger, as well as troubled personal relationships also may contribute to the development of disordered eating patterns. Likewise, major life transitions, the presence of other coping behaviours such as gambling, the presence of another psychiatric disorder such as clinical depression, and alcohol or drug abuse are associated with the onset of eating disorders.

There may be biochemical imbalances associated with eating disorders. The imbalances found in certain brain chemicals called neurotransmitters also are found in people suffering from depression. Neurotransmitters such as serotonin and norepinephrine control appetite, mood, alertness and sleeping patterns. Low levels of these chemicals may explain the link between eating disorders and depressive illness, as well as why people exhibit abnormal and seemingly illogical eating patterns. However, researchers still are not sure whether neurotransmitter imbalances are the cause of eating disorders or the result of the poor nutrition these disorders bring.

Treatments

Eating disorders are most successfully treated when detected in their early stages. *Anorexia nervosa* may not be detected until victims become seriously underweight, and *bulimia nervosa* victims can go on for years without anyone knowing about their disease. Fortunately, increasing awareness of the dangers of eating disorders has led more people to seek early help. According to the APA, simply restoring a person to normal weight or temporarily ending the binge-purge cycle does not address the underlying emotional problems that are caused, or are exacerbated by, the abnormal eating behaviour.

Treatment of eating disorders focuses on correcting the patient's distorted body image, improving self-confidence and self-esteem, treating any underlying depression, establishing normal eating habits and preventing relapse. Many victims can successfully be treated in out-patient programmes; however, in critical cases, hospitalisation is necessary.

A treatment plan will include a combination of physical interventions as well as individual, group or family psychotherapy, cognitive therapy, behaviour therapy and medications. To accomplish this level of treatment, a team approach is employed.

Medications are commonly prescribed for eating disorder patients. These medications, which regulate the body's level of neurotransmitters, can bring about improved self-esteem and a sense of control, as well as markedly reduce binge-and-purge behaviour in bulimics. Currently, the drug Prozac, a serotonin reuptake inhibitor which recently won the Food and Drug Administration's approval for use in treating *bulimia nervosa*, is the only drug specifically approved for the eating disorder.

The length of treatment for eating disorders varies, but it can take as long as five years. Success rates for treatment are difficult to estimate because continued treatment does not necessarily mean that the treatment is not working. Despite the complexities of treating eating disorders, sufferers have an excellent chance for complete recovery, especially if the illness is recognised early.

REFERENCES

Berg, F., 'Nondiet movement gains strength', *Obesity and Health* 6:85-90, 1992.

Bowen, D.J. et al., 'Influences on eating patterns of change to a lowfat diet, *JADA* 93:1309-1311, 1993.

Edwards, Sally, *Sally Edwards' Heart Zone Training: Exercise Smart, Stay Fit, And Live Longer*, Holbrook, MA: Adams Publishing, 1996.

Fletcher, Anne, *Thin for Life*, Shelburne, VT: Chapters Publishing, 1994.

Foreyt, J.P. and G. K. Goodrick, 'Weight management without dieting', *Nutrition Today* 28 (2): 4-9, 1993.

Hoeger, Werner and Sharon Hoeger, *Lifetime Physical Fitness And Wellness*, Englewood, CO: Morton Publishing, 1992.

Kingsbury, B., *Full Figure Fitness: A Program for Teaching Overweight Adults*, Champaign, IL: Life Enhancement Publications, 1993.

Oil That Heals: A Physicians Successes With Caster Oil Treatments, Mcgarey, William A. Paperback ISBN: 0876043082.

Oil-Protein Diet Cookbook, Budwig, Johanna Paperback ISBN: 0969527225.

Omega 3 Oils, Rudin, Donald Paperback ISBN: 0895297213.

Omega Diet, Wills, Judith Paperback ISBN: 074727195X.

Omega Diet: The Lifesaving Nutritional Program Based On The Diet Of The Island Of Crete, Simopoulos, Artemis P. Paperback ISBN: 0060930233.

Organic Living, Van Straten, Michael Hardcover/Clothcover ISBN: 0875969305.

Scott K. Powers Stephen L. Dodd, *Total Fitness: Exercise, Nutrition, and Wellness*, 1999.

4

Child Nutrition and Physical Activity

The fitness level of urban children today is much lesser than that it was a generation ago. Presently, they show signs of many severe diseases. Inactive children, when compared with active children, weigh more, have higher blood pressure and lower levels of heart-protective high-density lipoproteins. Even though heart attack and stroke are rare in children, evidence suggests that the process leading to those conditions begins in childhood.

These days at least half of youth do not engage in physical activity that promotes long-term health, that less than 50 per cent of primary and secondary schools offer daily PT classes, and that most classes were unlikely to foster lifelong physical activity. A fitness testing programme in the USA sponsored by the Chrysler Fund Amateur Athletic Union tracks fitness among 9.7 million youngster's between the ages of six and 17, and shows that children are getting slower in endurance running and are getting weaker. Since 1980 there has been a 10 per cent drop off on scores for distance runs and an 11 per cent decline in youngsters who achieved at least a satisfactory score on the entire test.

As many as one in five children between the ages of six and 17 are overweight. From 1963 to 1980 obesity increased 54 per cent among children six to 11 and 39 per cent in adolescents 12 to 17. 14.2 million girls and 12.8 million boys age

19 and under have serum cholesterol levels of 170 mg or higher. High serum cholesterol is most prevalent among African-American girls of all ages. An estimated 2.1 million adolescents aged 12 to 17 are smokers. Nine million American children under the age of five live with at least one smoker and are exposed to second-hand smoke for virtually the whole day. It is estimated that 3,000 American young people become smokers every day.

Inactive children are more likely to become inactive adults. Healthful lifestyle training should begin in childhood to promote improved cardiovascular health in adult life. The following good health practices should be promoted among children:

a) regular physical activity
b) a low-fat, low-cholesterol diet after the age of two
c) smoking prevention
d) appropriate weight for height
e) regular paediatric medical check-ups

Physical inactivity has been established as a major risk factor for the development of coronary artery disease. It also contributes to other risk factors including obesity, high blood pressure and a low level of HDL cholesterol. Even modest levels of physical activity are beneficial. Physical activity helps build and maintain healthy bones, muscles and joints. In addition, physically active children enjoy other health benefits, such as:

a) weight control
b) lower blood pressure
c) improved psychological well-being
d) a tendency to be more physically active as adults.

Regular physical activity in adulthood reduces the risk of heart disease. A healthy level of physical, activity requires regular participation in activities that increase energy expenditure above resting levels. An active child participates in physical education classes, plays sports, performs regular household chores, spends recreational time outdoors and regularly travels by foot or bicycle. Health professionals who make exercise recommendations for children should consider the child's age, gender and inclination toward activity. Some points to remember are:

a) Regular walking, bicycling and outdoor play; use of playgrounds and gymnasiums; and interaction with other children.
b) Less than two hours per day watching television or videotapes.
c) Weekly participation in age-appropriate organised sports, lessons, clubs or sandlot games.
d) Daily school or day-care physical education that includes at least 20 minutes of coordinated large muscle exercise.
e) Access to school buildings and community facilities that enable safe participation in physical activity.
f) A range of extracurricular programmes in schools and community recreation centres to meet the needs and interests of specific, populations, such as racial and ethnic minority groups, females, persons with disabilities and low-income groups.
g) Opportunities for physical activity that are fun, increase confidence in participating in physical activity, and involve friends and peers.
h) Regular family outings that involve walking, cycling, swimming or other recreational activities.
i) Positive role modelling for a physically active lifestyle by parents, physicians and school personnel.

Physical activity is important for all children, including those who are less coordinated. Physical activity may be particularly helpful for children with a weight problem in relation to both their physical and psychological well-being.

Healthy children, when in an environment conducive to physical activity, will be active. Emphasis should be placed on play and on activities that the child enjoys, that are consistent with the child's skill level, and that can be accomplished given the family's personal resources and interests.

Children are remarkably able to adjust their levels of activity to their individual capability. Maximum heart rate in healthy children is about 200 beats per minute, and there is no need to arbitrarily restrict them to lower heart rates. Therefore, taking target heart rates in healthy children is neither recommended nor necessary. In children with congenital or acquired cardiovascular diseases, there is no formula for calculating target heart rate. That is because the heart rates differ between individuals, depending on their cardiovascular condition. Exercise testing by a paediatric cardiologist can help determine the child's exercise capabilities, but there are no across-the-board recommendations.

Nutritionists have recognised the importance of establishing healthful nutrition practices during childhood and early adolescence. From birth to two years, a period characterised by rapid growth, gains in weight and height are the primary indices of nutritional status. Breast-feeding is encouraged for at least the first four to six months of life for nutritional as well as immunological benefits to the infant.

Among the most common nutritional disorders during infancy is iron deficiency anaemia, which is routinely screened for through blood tests of haemoglobin or haematocrit. Solid foods are usually introduced about four to six months of age, particularly iron-fortified cereals, to help prevent this problem. Other foods such as strained fruits and vegetables, and fruit juice are gradually introduced, until by about 12 months of age when most babies are eating small, tender table foods.

In children under two years of age, dietary fat plays a key role in the formation vital nerve and brain tissues. Health professionals do not recommend feeding fat-reduced foods to children of this age. Infants should never be put to bed with a bottle of milk formula, or other liquid to help guard against developing nursing bottle caries.

Recommendations of nutrients for children over the age of two differ little from those for adults. However, the recommendations are designed to promote optimal growth and development and, therefore, may not be restrictive as those for adults. A wide variety of foods, rich in essential nutrients necessary for growing bodies, form the basis of recommendations. Carbohydrate-rich grain foods, fruits and vegetables are necessary to supply vitamins, minerals, fibre and energy vital to good health. Adequate amounts of dairy products, lean meats, fish, poultry, eggs, dry beans and nuts also provide nutrients that contribute to proper growth and development.

Between the ages of 6-12, youngsters will grow to an average of one to two feet and almost double in weight. Diminished weight-for-height may be indicative of acute under-nutrition; a decreased height-for-age may suggest chronic under-nutrition. Such growth failure may be due to malnutrition, psychosocial deprivation, eating disorders, underlying chronic disease, infection or other factors. While children often have definite food likes and dislikes, nutritionists recommend parents make available a wide variety of foods and encourage tasting new foods in small quantities without forcing the issue.

Adolescents need extra-nutrients to support the adolescent growth spurt, which begins in girls at ages 10 or 11, reaches its peak at age 12 and is completed at about 15. In boys, it begins at 12 or 13 years of age, peaks at 14 and ends at about 19. In addition to other nutrients, adequate amounts of iron and calcium are particularly important as the body undergoes this intensive growth period. From ages 11 to 24 years, both males and females are encouraged to consume a calcium-rich diet in order to help ensure adequate calcium deposition in the bones during the age at which peak bone mass is attained. This may help reduce the incidence of osteoporosis in later years. By eating at least three servings daily from the milk, yogurt and cheese group, the recommended calcium intake can be achieved.

Teens' caloric needs vary depending on their growth rate, degree of physical maturation, body composition and activity level. Overweight is one of the most serious nutrition problems of adolescents. Eating disorders also are common among teens, whose food choices are often influenced by social pressure to achieve cultural ideals of thinness, gain peer acceptance, or assert independence from parental authority. According to the US National Centre for Health Statistics, one in 100 females between the ages of 12 and 18 has anorexia nervosa, a disorder causing people to severely limit their food intake.

Children and teens should eat at least three meals a day, to meet energy needs throughout the day. Eating breakfast affects both cognitive and physical performance; that is, if a child eats breakfast, he or she may be more alert in school and better able to learn and perform sports or other physical activities. Snacks also form an integral part of meal patterns for children and teens. Young children generally cannot eat large quantities at one sitting and get hungry long before the next regular meal-time. Mid-morning and mid-afternoon snacks are generally advised for this age. Fast-growing, active teens may have tremendous energy needs. Even though their regular meals can be substantial, they still may need snacks to supply energy between meals and to meet their daily nutrient needs.

CHILD OBESITY

Nowadays, childhood obesity is becoming one important physical problem. Data from the US National Health and Nutrition Examination Survey indicate that approximately 21 per cent of American adolescents between the ages of 12 and 19 can be described as overweight. Studies show that 20 to 40 per cent of American youngsters are physically unfit. Only a small percentage of obese children may attribute their problem to endocrine disorder or other underlying physical problems. While health professionals acknowledge the importance of a balanced diet, they rarely recommend severely restricting calories for overweight children. They do, however, stress the importance of increasing exercise and physical activity as a lifelong approach to weight management and overall good health and quality of life. Dietary guidelines also encourage children aged two and over to limit their consumption of dietary fat to 30 per cent or less of calories and saturated fat to ten per cent or less of calories.

The 1995 revision of the *Dietary Guidelines for Americans* includes the recommendation, "Balance the foods you eat with physical activity. Maintain your weight." In addition, the *Surgeon General's Report on Physical Activity and Health* released in 1996, recommends encouragement of physical activity behaviours among children and adolescents on the assumption that these behaviours will translate into adulthood. The US Centres for Disease Control and Prevention recommend that "Every American adult should accumulate 30 minutes or more of moderate-intensity physical activity over the course of most, preferably all, days of the week."

These reports present opportunities to promote physical activity messages as part of a healthful lifestyle for both children and adults alike. In addition to diminishing potential health problems, moderate physical activity provides more flexibility for consumers to expand their food choices. With increased energy expenditure, children and adolescents, as well as adults, can enhance the amount and variety of foods that can be consumed in a nutritious and satisfying diet.

The most common causes of child obesity are genetic factors, lack of physical activity, unhealthy eating patterns, or a combination of these factors. In rare cases, a medical problem, such as an endocrine disorder, may cause a child to become overweight. Your physician can perform a careful physical exam and some blood tests, to rule out this type of problem.

Children whose parents or brothers or sisters are overweight may be at an increased risk of becoming overweight themselves. Although weight problems run in families, not all children with a family history of obesity will be overweight. Genetic factors play a role in increasing the likelihood that a child will be overweight, but shared family behaviours such as eating and activity habits also influence body weight.

A child's total diet and his/her activity level both play an important role in determining a child's weight. The increasing popularity of television, computer and video games contributes to children's inactive lifestyles. A doctor is the best person to determine whether your child has a weight problem. Physicians will measure your child's weight and height to determine if your child's weight is within a healthy range. A physician will also consider your child's age and growth patterns to determine whether your child is overweight.

Assessing overweight in children is difficult because children grow in unpredictable spurts. For example, it is normal for boys to have a growth spurt in weight and catch up in height later. It is best to let your child's doctor determine whether your child will grow into a normal weight. If your doctor finds that your child is overweight, he or she may ask you to make some changes in your family's eating and activity habits.

The most important things you can do to help overweight children is to let them know that they are okay whatever their weight. Children's feelings about themselves often are based on their parents' feelings about them. If you accept your children at any weight, they will be more likely to accept and feel good about themselves. It is also important to talk to your children about weight, allowing them to share their concerns with you. Your child probably knows better than anyone else that he/she has a weight problem. For this reason, overweight children need support, acceptance, and encouragement from their parents. Parents should try not to set children apart because of their weight, but focus on gradually changing their family's physical activity and eating habits.

Family involvement helps to teach everyone healthful habits and does not single out the overweight child. Regular physical activity, combined with healthy eating habits, is the most efficient and healthful way to control your weight. It is also an important part of a healthy lifestyle. Some simple ways to increase your family's physical activity include the following:

a) Be a role model for your children. If your children see that you are physically active and have fun, they are more likely to be active and stay active for the rest of their lives.
b) Plan family activities that provide everyone with exercise and enjoyment, like walking, dancing, biking, or swimming.
c) Be sensitive to your child needs. Overweight children may feel uncomfortable about participating in certain activities. It is important to help your child find physical activities that they enjoy and that are not embarrassing or too difficult.
d) Reduce the amount of time you and your family spend in sedentary activities such as watching TV or playing video games.
e) Become more active throughout your day and encourage your family to do so as well.

FOOD GUIDE PYRAMID

The *Food Guide Pyramid* was put forth by USDA in 1992. No matter what your age—from two years and over—or your lifestyle, the pyramid can be your personal guide to healthful eating. It offers simple, practical advice to help you make choices that are consistent with the seven dietary guidelines. They are:

a) Eat a variety of foods.

b) Maintain a healthy weight.

c) Choose a diet low in fat, saturated fat and cholesterol.

d) Choose a diet with plenty of vegetables, fruits and grain products.

e) Use sugars only in moderation.

f) Use salt and sodium only in moderation.

g) If you drink alcoholic beverages, do so in moderation.

The pyramid encourages the basic principles of a healthful diet: variety, balance and moderation.

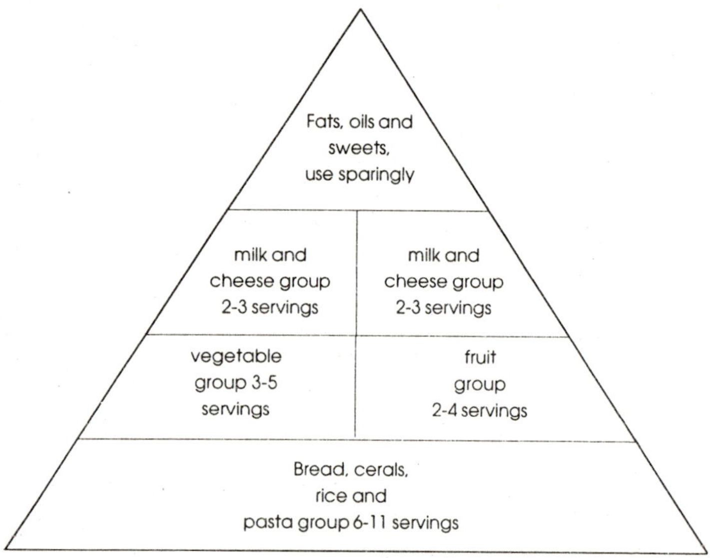

Fig. 4.1. Food guide pyramid

No single food supplies all the nutrients you need. A varied diet includes many different foods from the pyramid's five major food groups which together meet nutritional recommendations. A balanced diet incorporates appropriate amounts of foods from all five food groups every day, providing needed calories and nutrients. Your age, sex and physical activity level make difference in the number of servings needed to maintain a well-balanced diet.

Carefully selecting foods and beverages helps you control calories and the total amount of fat, saturated fat, cholesterol, salt, sugars and, if consumed, alcoholic beverages. This allows more flexibility to enjoy the variety of foods available.

You can adapt the pyramids advice to match your personal tastes and nutritional needs. In fact, the pyramid can be the food selection guide to meet differing needs of each family member, ages two and over. It may even help liven up your diet by expanding your food choices.

To make the most of the pyramid, you need to know what counts as a serving.

Food group	*Serving size*
Bread, Cereal, Pasta	1 slice bread, 1 ounce ready-to-eat cereal, 1/2 cup cooked cereal, rice or pasta.
Vegetable	1 cup raw, leafy vegetables, 1/2 cup cooked or chopped raw vegetables, 3/4 cup vegetable juice.
Fruit	1 medium apple, banana or orange, 1/2 cup chopped, cooked, or canned fruit, 3/4 cup fruit juice.
Milk, yogurt and cheese	1 cup milk or yogurt, $1_{1/2}$ ounces natural cheese, 2 ounces processed cheese.
Meat, poultry, fish, eggs and nuts	2 - 3 ounces cooked lean meat, poultry or fish Foods which count as 1 ounce of meat: 1/2 cup cooked dry beans, 1 egg, 2 tablespoons peanut butter, 1/3 cup nuts.

The range of servings of each food group in the pyramid offers lots of flexibility. The right amount for you depends on your age, sex, body size and activity level. The table below shows how many servings of each major food group can be included at different caloric levels. Pre-school children need the same variety of foods as older family members do, but may need less than 1,600 calories.

Table 4.1
Sample food plan for a day

	1,600 calories For many sedentary women and some older adults	*2,200 calories Most children teenage girls, active women and many sedentary men*	*2,800 calories Teenage boys, active men and some very active women*
Bread group	6	9	11
Fruit group	2	3	4
Vegetable group	3	4	5
Milk group	2-3*	2-3**	2-3**
Meat group	5 ounces	6 ounces	7 ounces

* Pregnancy and breast-feeding may require more calories.

** Women who are pregnant or breast-feeding, teenagers, and young adults to age 24 need three servings.

Healthful eating doesn't mean giving up foods and beverages you like best. Just learn how to balance your food choices. You can fit in your traditional favourites and enjoy your meals and snacks while still promoting your good health. Focus on foods such as pasta, rice and wholegrain and enriched breads and cereals, vegetables, fruits, low fat dairy foods, lean meats, poultry, fish and legumes. These foods provide the framework for a healthful diet.

a) Control calories and fat in food selection and preparation. For example, broil, roast, steam or stir-fry your favourite cut of lean meat, poultry without skin, or fish.

b) Modify traditional recipes to cut back on fat, saturated fat, cholesterol, added sugars and/or sodium. For example, try substituting plain, low fat yogurt for sour cream in dips or spreads, or use two egg whites or an egg substitute instead of one whole egg in baked foods.

c) Read food labels when you shop. The nutrition facts panel can help you compare the calories, fat, saturated fat, cholesterol, sodium and other nutrients in foods.

d) Eat smaller amounts of the richer foods you like.

No foods are good or bad for you; it is your total diet that counts. So there is no need to eliminate any one food. Every food can fit into a varied, moderate and balanced diet. Mixed, or combination, foods can wrap ingredients from two or more food groups into one food. Mixed foods help you meet the recommendations of the pyramid, while adding flavour and enjoyment to your meals. Consider a chicken burrito. Two ounces of shredded, broiled chicken offers two ounces from the meat group. A soft tortilla counts as one bread group serving. Three tablespoons (3/4 ounce) of low or reduced fat monterey jack cheese is equal to 1/2 milk group serving. And 1/4 cup chopped tomato and 1/2 cup shredded lettuce is equal to one vegetable group serving.

Many of the new food choices are really varieties of traditional favourites, yet they have fewer calories, and less fat, saturated fat, cholesterol, sugars or sodium. Fat-free mayonnaise and salad dressings and reduced fat sour cream are some examples. Like traditional foods, these foods are still part of the food guide pyramid. So count them toward your food group servings. For instance, reduced-fat cheese belongs in the milk group. Choose these modified foods as one way to moderate the calories, fat, cholesterol, sugars and sodium in your food choices. Use the nutrition facts panel on food labels to compare nutrients in these new foods with their traditional counterparts.

After you have made progress in moderating your intake of fat, sugars and calories, you can personalise your pyramid even further through trade offs! But what does 'trading off' mean? When you choose a food that is higher in fat, sugars or salt, select other foods that are lower in these ingredients to balance your total diet. Trading off gives flexibility. You can eat some, foods with more fat or more sugars, including those from the pyramid tip, and still consume a healthful diet. The key is to balance how much of these foods you eat and how often you eat them.

The following changes can make it easier to include your favourite foods in your diet:

a) *Trading-off fat*: Save some fat by switching from regular mozzarella to reduced fat mozzarella. To save more fat, substitute low fat cottage or ricotta cheese for whole milk ricotta. Then spend some of the fat savings on a little margarine to make crusty Italian garlic bread. Use fat-free dressing on your salad at lunch. For a snack later on, enjoy some guacamole dip with low fat crackers or raw vegetables. Grill or bake chicken breasts for dinner and remove the skin for more fat savings.

b) *Trading-off sugars*: Top your breakfast waffles with fresh berries instead of syrup. You'll save on sugars and calories and get more nutrients and fibre, too. Save the sugars for a sweet snack or beverage in the afternoon. For your mid-morning snack, choose fruit yogurt with low-calorie sweetener. Then spend your sugar savings on some jelly or honey with a roll later in the day. Use the nutrition facts panel on food labels to help make trade-offs.

Sugars added to foods enhance taste and perform other important functions in baking, cooking and preserving foods.

While they provide calories, they contribute few other nutrients. The amount of fat and sugars you eat over time is what counts. When you trade-off, do not panic if you over-indulge on one day; simply cut back on fat and sugars the next day.

Like sound eating habits, regular physical activity is a part of a healthy lifestyle. Among its many benefits, exercise burns calories and can help you manage your weight. Increasing your physical activity can also allow you to eat more calories without weight gain. Choose those extra calories mainly from the five major food groups. The only way to lose weight is to use more calories than you consume. Apply the same principles—variety, balance and moderation—to both food choices and exercise. Always check with your physician before beginning any exercise programme. Enjoy many different activities to exercise different muscles, including your heart.

Since different activities have different benefits, balance your exercise pattern. For overall fitness, you need exercises that build cardiovascular endurance, muscular strength, bone strength and flexibility. Exercise to keep fit, without overdoing. You don't need a heavy work-out everyday. Although exercise recommendations vary, health experts do advise 30 minutes or more of moderate exercise in your daily routine, most days, of the week.

To keep fit, you need to make balanced food choices for a lifetime. Start building your personal pyramid now.

a) Modify your food choices gradually. That may be easier than overhauling your whole diet at one time.

b) Choose foods each day from the five major food groups. Build your pyramid from the bottom up with plenty of grains, fruits and vegetables. How might your dinner plate look? Divide your plate in four sections. Fill three sections with vegetables, fruits and grains and the fourth with a lower fat choice from the meat group. Then add a fifth menu item—a glass of low fat milk.

c) Make moderation, not elimination, your goal. Eat foods lower in fat and sugars more often than those which have more.

d) Go for variety within the food groups. Take your taste buds on an adventure by trying new foods. Besides the nutritional benefits, variety adds interest to meals and snacks.

e) Consider your lifestyle and how many calories you need daily. Then, from each food group, eat enough servings—at least the minimum daily—to reach or keep your healthy weight.

The beauty of the food guide pyramid truly is its flexibility. As you grow older or your lifestyle, health condition or activity level changes, simply adjust how many servings of each food group you eat.

Teaching healthy eating practices early will help children approach eating with the right attitude that food should be enjoyed and is necessary for growth, development, and for energy to keep the body running. The best way to begin is to learn more about children's nutritional needs by reading or talking with a health professional and then to offer them some healthy options, allowing your children to choose what and how much they eat. Here are some ways to help your child develop good attitudes about eating.

a) *Don't place your child on a restrictive diet*: Children should never be placed on a restrictive diet to lose weight, unless a doctor supervises one for medical reasons. Limiting what children eat may be harmful to their health and interfere with their growth and development. To promote proper growth and development and prevent overweight, parents should offer a wide variety of foods from each of the food groups displayed in the food guide pyramid. It applies to healthy people aged two years and older and illustrates the importance of balance among food groups in a daily eating pattern. Select most of your daily servings of food from the food groups that are the largest in the picture and closest to the bottom of the pyramid.

b) Most of the foods in your diet should come from the grain products group (6-11 servings), the vegetable group (three/five servings), and the fruit group (two/four servings).

c) Your diet should include moderate amounts of foods from the milk group (two/three servings) and the meat and beans group (two/three servings).

d) Foods that provide few nutrients and are high in fat and sugars should be used sparingly. Fat should not be restricted in the diets of children younger than two years of age.

e) Carefully cut down on the amount of fat in your family's diet. Reducing fat is a good way to cut calories without depriving your child of nutrients. Simple ways to cut the fat in your family's diet include eating low-fat or non-fat dairy products, poultry without skin, and lean meats, and low-fat or fat-free breads and cereals. Making small changes to the amount of fat in your family's diet is a good way to prevent excess weight gain in children: however, major efforts to change your child's diet should be supervised by a health professional. In addition, fat should not be restricted in the diets of children younger than two years of age. After that age, children should gradually adopt a diet that contains no more than 30 per cent of calories from fat by the time the child is about 5 years old.

f) Don't overlay restrict sweets or treats. While it is important to be aware of the fat, salt, and sugar content of the foods you serve, all foods—even those that are high in fat or sugar—have a place in the diet, in moderation.

g) Guide your family's choices rather than dictate foods. Make a wide variety of healthful foods available in the house. This practice will help your children learn how to make healthy food choices.

h) Encourage your child to eat slowly. A child can detect hunger and fullness better when eating slowly.

i) Eat meals together as a family as often as possible. Try to make meal-times pleasant with conversation and sharing, not a time for scolding or arguing. If meal-times are unpleasant, children may try to eat faster to leave the table as soon as possible.

j) Involve children in food shopping and preparing meals. These activities offer parents hints about children's food preferences, teach children about nutrition, and provide children with a feeling of accomplishment. In addition, children may be more willing to eat or try foods that they help prepare.

k) Plan for snacks. Continuous snacking may lead to overeating, but snacks that are planned at specific times during the day can be part of a nutritious diet, without spoiling a child's appetite at meal-times. You should make snacks as nutritious as possible, without depriving your child of occasional chips or cookies, especially at parties or other social events.

Discourage eating meals or snacks while watching TV. Try to eat only in designated areas of your home, such as the dining room or kitchen. Eating in front of the TV may make it difficult to pay attention to feelings of fullness, and may lead to overeating.

Try not to use food to punish or reward your child. Withholding food as a punishment may lead children to worry that they will not get enough food. For example, sending children to bed without any dinner may cause them to worry that they will go hungry. As a result, they may try to eat whenever they get a chance. Similarly, when foods, such as sweets, are used as a reward, children may assume that these foods are better or more valuable than other foods.

Make sure your child's meals outside the home are balanced. Find out more about your school lunch programme, or pack your child's lunch to include a variety of foods. If your efforts at home are unsuccessful in helping your child reach a healthy weight and your physician determines that your child's health is at risk unless he/she loses weight steadily, you may want to consider a formal treatment programme. Look for the following characteristics when choosing a weight-control programme for your child. The programme should:

a) staffed with a variety of health professionals. The best programmes may include RDs, exercise physiologists, paediatricians or family physicians, and psychiatrists or psychologists.

b) perform a medical evaluation of the child. Before being enrolled in a programme, your child's weight, growth, and health should be reviewed by a physician. During enrolment, your child's weight, growth, and health should be monitored by a health professional at regular intervals.

c) focus on the whole family, not just the overweight child.

d) adapted to the specific age and capabilities of the child. Programmes for four-year-olds are different from those developed for children eight or twelve years of age in terms of degree of responsibility of the child and parents.

e) focus on behavioural changes.

f) teach the child how to select a variety of foods in appropriate portions.

g) encourage daily activity and limit sedentary activity, such as watching TV.

h) include a maintenance programme and other support and referral resources to reinforce the new behaviours and to deal with underlying issues that contributed to overweight.

The overall goal of a successful treatment programme should be to help the whole family focus on making healthy changes to their eating and activity habits that they will be able to maintain throughout life.

An overweight child runs a higher chance of being an overweight adult and subsequently faces higher risk for heart disease, diabetes, cancer, arthritis and other diseases, and it is painfully clear that obesity during childhood needs to be prevented. At least one in five kids today is overweight, a 50 per cent jump in the last two decades. As our children grow heavier, health professionals and parents alike want to know why and how to prevent it.

Research has identified a variety of factors that predict whether children will be physically active. Many of these factors form barriers against physical activity, and they must be recognised if efforts to increase physical activity are to be successful. Among these are time spent outdoors, which is affected by relatively innocuous issues such as the weather but also by more serious concerns such as children's safety. In addition, how a child thinks and feels about physical activity has a significant impact on his or her participation. Enjoying physical activity is perhaps the most powerful psychological influence, meaning fun and pleasure are the key to successful physical activity programmes.

A child's physical activity, self-efficacy, or confidence in his/her ability at sports, games and active play, is also crucial to developing a positive attitude about physical activity. Positive experiences go a long way toward building a child's confidence. Then there is the question of what everyone else is doing. According to Pate, social norms and influences are extremely powerful shapers of physical activity behaviour. Indeed, peer influences outrank parental influences as children grow older. But there is no ignoring the critical role of adult modelling and support in keeping kids active.

It is required that comprehensive guidelines are issued for school and community programmes to promote lifelong physical activity among young people. The guidelines should include recommendations covering varied aspects of school and community programmes. Perhaps the most important recommendation focuses on public policy. According to him, the challenge is to get the public and decision makers to take this seriously and to reinvest existing resources—perhaps invest new resources—in attacking the problem. There should be guidelines for a requirement of daily physical education in schools and comprehensive school health education.

There is also a need to modify the focus of physical education programmes. In physical education, the tradition has been to deal with physical skills, such as learning to play a sport. But physical education also needs to emphasise the behavioural skills associated with developing an active lifestyle, such as how to become less sedentary. Programmes that allow kids to be active at school are also important. After and outside of school, extracurricular activities need to be offered that appeal to all kids.

HEALTHY ATTITUDE OF TODAY'S KIDS

If a positive attitude is the first step to better health, today's kids are well on their way. Of the youngsters questioned in a new gallup survey in US, 97 per cent agree that a balanced diet is very important for good health, and 98 per cent agree that physical activity is too. Although they get an "A" for attitude, kids are not making the grade when it comes to understanding what constitutes good nutrition and exercising as much as they should. Developed by the American Dietetic Association (ADA) and the International Food Information Council (IFIC) in cooperation with the President's Council on Physical Fitness and Sports (PCPFS), the survey assessed the attitudes and behaviours of 410 children between the ages of nine and 15 regarding food, nutrition and physical activity.

The Gallup Organisation conducted the survey in late 1994 as a follow-up to a similar survey conducted in 1991. The survey found that kids are beginning to understand the basic tenets of healthy eating: variety, balance, and moderation. Nearly all (96 per cent) say they like eating different types of food. However, the youngsters surveyed also hold some misconceptions about nutrition despite the growing amount of nutrition information available. Nearly three-fourths (71 per cent) feel that their favourite foods are not good for them, a slight increase from the 1991 survey results.

Kids are changing today. Most kids do not eat three meals a day. Half of the respondents of the survey say they skip breakfast, and 20 per cent skip lunch. In addition, 18 per cent say they skip dinner, an increase of six percentage points in the last three years. More and more youngsters agree that snacks can be an important part of a healthy diet. Hurried lifestyles, coupled with the smaller portions kids eat, mean many youngsters are not able to sit down and eat a full meal.

Snacks are an important part of the diet because they help prevent between meal hunger and fatigue. Foods such as cheese, pretzels, fruit or cut raw vegetables are great snacks that help kids refuel throughout the day and are easy to carry in a back-pack or bag. More kids are eating the school lunch, according to the survey. More than two-thirds say they eat school lunches, and 29 per cent take their lunch to school. In 1991, 58 per cent said they ate the school's lunch, and 40 per cent brown bagged it.

Today's kids like being physically active. The most common reason kids gave for being active was because it is fun, and 78 per cent of those surveyed say they enjoy and look forward to participating in physical activity or sports. Furthermore, 80 per cent say they want to be more active in the coming year. When asked what activities they had engaged in during the last six months, the youngsters surveyed say playing outdoors (66 per cent), walking (62 per cent), jogging or running (59 per cent), riding a bicycle (58 per cent), and playing basketball (56 per cent). More than half of those surveyed say they either play outside or walk every day.

While the majority of kids are involved in a sport or specific activity, they may not be participating regularly in both moderate and vigorous activities. Moderate physical activities such as running or aerobic dancing should be included every other day. This can be achieved by making some basic changes. By changing a few habits, young people can significantly increase their physical activity levels and find that, in a short while, they feel and even look better. Walking or biking to a friends house instead of getting a ride is one possibility. Taking the stairs at the shopping mall instead of the escalator or elevator is another. Taking a 10-minute break every hour from studying or watching television to walk around the house or around the block or turn on a radio and dance will also improve health.

SCHOOLS AS ROLE MODELS

Schools play a pivotal role in moulding children's attitudes and behaviours about nutrition and physical activity. For example, schools and teachers are considered to be the major sources of nutrition information for 90 per cent of the respondents, and 60 per cent rate that information as very useful. Teachers are in the unique position of being able to tie the classroom into the lunch-room. Whether the subject is science, history, maths or home economics, all classes are a forum for children to learn about food, eating and nutrition.

School provides a place to get the exercise children need to develop properly. However, only one-third of all respondents report taking physical education class five days a week; another 38 per cent take it two or three days a week. Some schools are looking for other ways to incorporate physical activities into the class schedule. The survey found that, of those who said they do not attend PT, two-fifths (41 per cent) said they do participate in some type of physical activity in another class. Furthermore, 26 per cent of all the respondents say they attend an after school programme almost every day, while another 20 per cent do so two or three times a week.

Schools are the place, where children get their nutrition and physical activity information, where many receive at least one meal a day, and where most children are given a chance to be physically active. It is crucial that we as a society support our schools and continue offering the top-notch information and resources our children need for optimal growth and development.

Many parents wrongly assume that children are incapable of regulating their food intake, that children don't know the difference between hungry and full. Does the child know he needs some peas? No. Does a child know how much he wants to eat? Yes. Thus, the responsibility of parents is to provide the variety of foods children need and then allow them to obey their internal cues and eat as much or as little as they want.

If we are beginning to err in any direction, it is making eating into an issue of individual foods and individual nutrients. We are getting too micro-oriented when, in fact, eating is not just about food. Eating occasions are not only about limiting fat or getting enough of a certain vitamin. They also include talking about your day, engaging in discourse with people you like. If parents can focus on some of the pleasant things about eating, some of the food struggles may diminish.

Parents need to discriminate between a child who is possibly bored and one who is really hungry. Set some limits on what foods you will offer and when. If a child is hungry, offer something like a banana or raisins, even a cookie.

Parents have the responsibility to provide a variety of selections so that a sweet treat is just one of many foods offered in a day. Never let a kid have a sweet invested food, which can cause problems later on. Kids' stomachs are small. If you dilute the caloric density of the diet too much, the child won't be able to eat enough to satisfy his or her energy needs. Children need high-caloric snacks from time to time.

Parents who could not control their eating, who didn't stop eating when they were no longer hungry, had children who also had problems controlling the amount they ate. This may indicate that children are modelling their parents' behaviour or that a genetic basis exists for these similarities within a family.

We know that differences between girls and boys exist, but we don't have a clear picture of the origins of those differences. If one places a girl and a boy in equal laboratory settings so that the child is making the decisions about eating, boys will regulate better than girls. It could mean there's a biological rationale for the difference. But considering what we know about our culture's values, the vigilance about women's eating habits and their figures, another interpretation could be that, as early as age three or four, mothers may be setting more limits on what daughters eat than they do on sons. What the parent really needs and wants is information about what the child had to eat before coming home to dinner. What is the best thing parents can do to avoid obesity in their children?

First, serve a variety of foods and let your kids see you eating them. It has been shown time and again that kids' food preferences are driven by what they eat most often. It is a matter of exposure. Children need to taste a new food eight to ten times before they will learn to accept it, if the parent hangs in there and does not give up after two or three rejections. Chances are the child will learn to like a wide variety of foods, even peas and carrots.

Second, get physical. Show kids how much fun it is to be physically active. Exercise is extremely important in maintaining one's health, and active parents inspire active kids. In fact, one of the best predictors of whether a child will be active is if the parents are. Dads seem to have particular influence, perhaps because they are often not around as much and therefore what they do is more noticeable. In fact, for the overweight child, the best thing a parent can do is to find a physical activity that the child likes, provide a healthy variety of food and place less stress on food and eating.

According to the third National Health and Nutrition Examination Survey (NHANES) of US obesity among six-to-17-year olds more than doubled between 1988 and 1991. Richard P. Troiano, Ph.D., R.D., and colleagues at the National Centre for Health Statistics studied 2,290 children and compared their results with earlier NHANES surveys. They found that during the 1960s and 1970s, the prevalence of overweight generally was steady among adolescents and rose slowly in children. But the greatest increase in overweight prevalence occurred between the mid-1970s and early 1990s. According to the study reported in *Archives of Paediatrics and Adolescent Medicine*, 22 per cent of children and adolescents fit the criteria for overweight, up from 15 per cent in the previous survey. Troiano noted that overweight may be a part of normal growth, as young adolescents experience rapid changes which require time for their bodies to adjust.

Although some overweight youths will lose their excess weight as they mature and develop, many may go on to become overweight adults. This implies an increased need for treatment of morbidities associated with overweight in the near and distant future. Total caloric and fat intake of the children varied little across the years. Thus, finding the root of the overweight problem remains a challenge. Dietary treatment for obesity has been largely ineffective in children and is complicated by the need to avoid interference with their optimal growth and development. Attempts to increase physical activity for children and adolescents may be a promising avenue in this effort.

Judy Dodd, M.S., R.D., a counsellor in child and adolescent nutrition and former president of the *American Dietetic Association*, concurs: "One of the basic principles of weight loss and maintenance is to use the same number of calories taken in. Kids lead a much more sedentary life than ever before. They don't have the opportunity or the interest in playing or being active." The new data may be the call to action that adults and children have needed. "All adults from parents and teachers to coaches and celebrities influence kids' choices and decisions. This is the wake-up call we need to encourage our kids to get up and move", said Dodd.

During preschool and childhood years, foods should not be eliminated or restricted because of the fat content, according to a joint working group of the Canadian Paediatric Society and Health and Welfare Canada. At the American Dietetic Association's Annual Meeting in October, Canadian and US nutritionists examined paediatric dietary guidelines and identified universal ways to improve youngsters' eating habits.

Recently, both American and Canadian dietary guidelines for children two years of age and older recommend 30 per cent or less of total calories from dietary fat; saturated fat should contribute 10 per cent or less of calories. This guideline is often referred to as the "30/10" approach. Most American health authorities believe children who adopt such dietary guidelines at a young age have a better chance of continuing sound eating habits as they mature, and that such children will have a reduced risk of heart disease. Many Canadian experts, however, stress that too little fat in children's diets may inhibit their proper growth and development. Rather, the emphasis should be on providing an adequate energy intake, with a gradual lowering of fat intake during adolescence.

The Canadian Working Group compared information on nutritional needs for paediatric growth and development with evidence linking diet and heart disease among adults. They concluded that the most important dietary issue for children is providing proper nutrients for optimal growth and development. Eliminating or restricting foods is not prudent since young children tend to consume a limited range of foods. They also noted that preferences and habits change drastically during the early years. Therefore, it is impossible to predict whether lifelong eating habits will improve with the next generation.

According to AAP, no evidence suggests that following the 30/10 recommendation will adversely affect proper growth and development. Furthermore, preliminary results show significant disease risk reduction can be achieved in youngsters who follow the low-fat guidelines. The AAP encourages parents to use the 30/10 ratio as a guideline, and to introduce the concepts of balance, variety and moderation to their children as they try new foods. This approach underscores the importance of not eating too much of any one type of food or nutrient, so that by the time youngsters reach adolescence the transition to a lower-fat diet will be easier.

In recent decades, public health authorities have stressed the need to modify children's diets to reduce their risk of chronic diseases. But several conference speakers labelled the link between children's diets and chronic illness "tenuous" and in need of further study.

REFERENCES

Berg, F., 'Nondiet movement gains strength', *Obesity and Health* 6:85-90, 1992.

Cooper, Robert K., *Health And Fitness Excellence*, Boston: Houghton Mifflin, 1989.

Edwards, Sally, *Sally Edwards' Heart Zone Training: Exercise Smart, Stay Fit, And Live Longer*, Holbrook, MA: Adams Publishing, 1996.

Jerrold S. Greenberg George B. Dintiman Barbee Myers Oakes, *Wellness: Creating a Life of Health and Fitness*, 1997.

Obesity (Lucent Overview Series), Akers, Charlene Library binding, hard cover book ISBN: 1560066628.

Obesity Sourcebook (Health Reference Series), Caldwell, Wilma (eds., Kimball, Chad T. (eds.) Hardcover ISBN: 0780803337.

Obesity: Pathophysiology, Psychology, and Treatment, (Chapman and Hall Series in Clinical Nutrition), Blackburn, George L., Kanders, Beatrice S. (eds.), Hardcover ISBN: 041298461X.

Omichinski, Linda and Kathleen Harrison,'Nondiet Weight Management: A Lifestyle Approach to Health and Fitness', San Marcos, *Nutrition Dimension,* 1995.

Randall R. Cottrell James T. Girvan James F. McKenzie, *Principles and Foundations of Health Promotion and Education*, 1999.

Rebecca J. Donatelle, *Health: The Bas ics,* 2001.

5

Adult Nutrition and Physical Activity

At the dawn of the new millennium, concerns about adult nutrition differ significantly from those of earlier years. Prior to World War II, the main nutritional problems stemmed from a lack of sufficient food or variety of foods. Nutrition scientists of that era focused on defining essential nutrients, primarily vitamins, in order to outline the minimum food intake necessary for good health. As society became more affluent, however, nutritional concerns changed from the effects of too little food or nutrients to an overabundance of food or certain nutrients.

Epidemiological and laboratory studies demonstrated a link between dietary excesses and chronic diseases such as coronary heart disease and cancer. These findings led to the development of dietary recommendations intended to reduce people's risk of chronic diseases. In the late 1970s, the Senate Select Committee on Nutrition and Human Needs of USA issued the dietary goals. Since then, various federal agencies have issued similar recommendations for achieving a healthy diet. Dietary recommendations developed by independent health organisations also indicate a general consensus among nutrition scientists regarding the role of diet in health and disease.

Modern dietary recommendations focus on ensuring an adequate intake of nutrients such as carbohydrates and fibre, while moderating others such as dietary fat, which may be linked to the development of chronic disease.

The recommendations are largely summed up in *Nutrition and Your Health: Dietary Guidelines for Americans*. This publication was first developed in 1980 by the US Department of Agriculture (USDA) and the Department of Health and Human Services for use in consumer nutrition education efforts with healthy Americans aged two years and older. The fourth edition issued in December 1995 advises:

a) Eat a variety of foods.
b) Balance the food you eat with physical activity—maintain or improve your weight.
c) Choose a diet with plenty of vegetables, fruits, and grain products.
d) Choose a diet low in fat, saturated fat and cholesterol.
e) Choose a diet moderate in sugars.
f) Choose a diet moderate in salt and sodium.
g) If you drink alcoholic beverages, do so in moderation.
h) These guidelines are reviewed every five years and was updated in the year 2000.

In 1992, the USDA put forth the food guide pyramid as a nutrition education tool to help put the *Dietary Guidelines for Americans* into action. The pyramid serves as a general guide for daily food choices. It includes specific recommendations for daily intake of five different food groups as well as guidelines for moderating intake of fat and sugars.

In US, the *Dietary Guidelines Alliance* was formed among health organisations, the food industry and the government to develop effective, consumer-focused messages to convey the *Dietary Guidelines for Americans.* "It's All About You" is a useable message campaign that translates the recommendations into simple, positive ways consumers can integrate these basic health principles into their lives. It consists of five core messages designed to motivate consumers into rethinking and positively changing their eating and activity routines, which are:

a) *Be realistic*: Make small changes over time in what you eat and the level of activity you do. After all, small steps work better than giant leaps.
b) *Be adventurous*: Expand your tastes to enjoy a variety of foods.
c) *Be flexible*: Go ahead and balance what you eat and the physical activity you do over several days. No need to worry about just one meal or one day.
d) *Be sensible*: Enjoy all foods, just do not overdo it.
e) *Be active*: Walk the dog, don't just watch the dog walk.

Healthy People 2000 was a national initiative of the US Department of Health and Human Services to improve the health of all Americans through prevention. It was driven by 300 specific national health promotion and disease prevention objectives targeted for achievement by the year 2000. The overall goals of the national initiative were to increase the span of healthy life, reduce health disparities among Americans and achieve access to preventive services. Nutrition is one of 22 priority areas in *Healthy People 2000*'s national health promotion and disease prevention objectives.

SOLUTIONS TO ELDERLY MALNUTRITION

Yet malnutrition is a serious health problem among the nation's elderly, according to a recent survey of health professionals specialising in elder care. The survey of 750 physicians, nurses and administrators of health care institutions found that one in four elderly patients is malnourished. One-half of all elderly hospital patients and 40 per cent of nursing home residents are believed to suffer from malnutrition. Elderly people are not getting proper nutrients because of deficiencies, excesses, or imbalances in food or diet, according to the survey sponsored by the Nutrition Screening Initiative (NSI), a coalition of more than 30 national medical, health and aging organisations.

To help educate dietitians and other health care professionals about the importance of elderly nutrition, the American Dietetic Association Foundation and the International Food Information Council Foundation have been sponsoring a seminar series, 'Better Eating for Better Aging,' in conjunction with various state dietetic associations.

Nutrition plays a significant role in the prevention of illness, as well as in treatment and recovery. Many elderly have unmet health needs, which affect their nutritional status. Many older people living alone have declining motor skills, making it difficult to shop for or cook food. Depression also can affect their nutritional status. To identify those at risk of malnutrition, nutrition screening should be routinely incorporated into medical examinations.

A nutrition screen can range from a simple review of weight, height, skin tone, diet, living conditions and behaviour, to blood tests and sophisticated assessment techniques. A self-administered checklist is available from NSI to spot eating problems, economic hardship and other conditions affecting nutritional status. Among the primary reasons many elderly become malnourished are losses in their senses of taste and smell. Without the simple pleasures of taste and smell, the overall quality of life is greatly reduced, especially for the elderly whose senses decline due to aging.

Declines in taste and smell usually begin around 60 years of age and become more pronounced in subsequent decade of life. Certain diseases and/or medications is prescribed for such conditions also can contribute to chemosensory losses. Thresholds, or the levels at which flavours are detected, are about 2.5 times higher in the elderly than in young college students. But the threshold for detecting fat in food is four times higher in the elderly, which can be problematic for many seniors following low-fat diets. People with higher thresholds for taste may have difficulty following a low-fat diet because they miss the mouthfeel contributed by fat and certain odour molecules, which are primarily fat soluble.

To increase consumption of lower-fat, nutrient dense foods, we should improve the taste by adding herbs, spices or flavour enhancers such as monosodium glutamate (MSG) Although scientists once believed there were only four taste sensations—sweet, salty, sour and bitter—new data suggest that there are many more tastes such as glutamate. This taste, known as *umami* to the Japanese, has been described by Westerners as brothy or meat-like. Elderly people may be unknowingly consuming large amounts of fat without being able to really perceive it. Yet MSG can be used in foods to help replace some of the mouthfeel normally contributed by fat, allowing older persons to enjoy their food while maintaining a nutritionally adequate, low-fat diet.

Adding glutamate to blended or table food improves appetite and reverses the effects of anorexia among the elderly in long-term care settings. MSG has been added to foods since the turn of the century and is classified by the Food and Drug Administration (FDA) as a Generally Recognised and Safe (GRAS) food ingredient. FDA is currently updating its review of MSG safety as part of its ongoing review of all GRAS ingredients, and is expected to issue a report next year.

There is no end in sight to our focus on the baby boom generation, even as we approach the 21st century. Baby boomers will be a key factor in the coming 'age-quake', when the elderly will comprise a much larger share of the population. In 1980, about one in 10 persons were 65 or older. By 2030, the 65 and older will number one in five. The first 'boomers' will reach age 65 in 2011. And more people will be living longer. According to most projections, tomorrow's 85-plus will be a fast growing group as the median age of death in the next century climbs to 84 years.

The needs of an aging population will shape every facet of society in the next century, including nutrition. The recently-revised Recommended Daily Allowances (RDAs) do not distinguish among older adults of various ages. There is just one set of RDAs for all adults over age 50. Most experts agree that the dietary needs of people in their 50s or 60s are different from people in their 70s and 80s.

VITAMIN REQUIREMENTS

There are generally recognised changes in dietary needs for the elderly. Many are related to loss of lean body mass and reduced level of activity. Less muscle tissue and lower expenditure of energy result in four need for reduced caloric intake. When eating less food, the elderly must be careful to select nutritious foods so that their diminished intake will provide the nutrients they need. In general, women require fewer calories, yet have nutrient requirements similar to men, and must be especially mindful of their food choices.

Normal changes associated with aging result in higher requirements for some nutrients such as vitamin D, which is necessary for proper calcium absorption. The elderly typically get less exposure to the sun and have reduced capacity for skin synthesis of vitamin D, a major source of this. Reduced intakes as well as lower absorption and metabolism of vitamin D and calcium are among the many factors related to loss of bone mineral. This leads to susceptibility to fractures and related problems, including morbidity and mortality.

The elderly also seem to require more vitamin B_6, and may be more sensitive to its depletion. Neurolgic and immunologic effects may become apparent, although they are reversible with supplementation. As many as 30 per cent of people at age 65 develop atrophic gastritis, the inability to produce stomach acid. This leads to impaired absorption of certain important nutrients, including folic acid, calcium, iron and vitamin B_{12}. He estimated that by the age of 80, up to 40 per cent of persons develop atrophic gastritis, which has a significant impact on the bio-availability of some key nutrients.

The elderly clear vitamin A from their blood and tissue more slowly, meaning they can be more susceptible to vitamin A toxicity. An over-supply of vitamin A could easily be harmful. Research into vitamins E and C, both antioxidants, may lead to new RDAs for the elderly one day. Vitamin E has shown a positive effect on the immune system in research at the USDA Centre. Whether vitamin E stimulates the immune system or prevents its decline is unclear. An increased chance of developing cataracts has been associated with low vitamin C intakes in research at the USDA Centre. Vitamin C's anti-oxidant properties may ward off potential damage by ultra-violet light, but the conclusion cannot yet be drawn.

Aging is generally associated with decline of the immune response, which may be linked with a cumulative, marginal deficiency of trace metals and vitamins. Of particular interest are zinc, B vitamins, iron and other trace metals. Medications for chronic disease can affect drug-nutrient interaction as well. These and other emerging ideas lead many to call for more definitive research into the nutritional needs of the elderly.

Elderly on low, fixed incomes are at greater risk of malnutrition. A lack of skills and knowledge about food preparation is another problem. The loneliness and despair felt by some elderly also contribute to loss of appetite. Somewhat striking is the significance of living arrangement, especially for men. Research has found a correlation between living alone and a poor quality diet.

Researches have speculated reasons for solitary older people, showing poor nutritional habits vary with gender. Men living alone are at particular risk because they are traditionally unaccustomed to planning, shopping and preparing for meals. On the other hand, women may feel unmotivated to prepare meals when there is no one to share them with. Some simple tips developed by the American Association of Retired Persons (AARP) may help the elderly who live alone. AARP suggests inviting a friend over to share a meal or having a standing date with a friend to eat out together weekly. Other tips include buying smaller food packages to reduce repetitious meals of leftovers, and setting the dining table attractively. AARP also recommends joining a nutrition programme at a community or senior centre.

Senses of taste and smell decline with age for a variety of reasons. The loss can result from disease, injury or drug, treatments, as well as from normal aging. Without the pleasure of eating, the overall quality of life for older people is greatly reduced. This can increase depression and stress, and lead to poor nutrition. In extreme cases, older people can become anorexic. A taste disorder can also cause poor digestion by altering salivary flow and intestinal motility.

Odour and flavour enhancers may become an important factor in developing special food products for the elderly. Gradual, steady loss of body water is a factor in aging, and older people more easily become dehydrated. This can be a major complicating factor in illness and negatively affects outcome. The reasons may be impaired renal, concentrating ability, causing excessive water to pass, and impaired sense of thirst.

In some studies, thirst-impaired seniors do not seek water, even when water is physically needed and available. Habit also influences water intake, as some elderly avoid the greater likelihood of urinary incontinence by drinking less water. It is important to find ways to overcome dehydration as a buffer in case of illness and as possible protection from the aging process. Finding a way to slow the aging process is a mythic quest, which has not yet been abandoned entirely.

Nutrition science is concentrating as never before on the special needs of older adults. The food industry is developing products and services of greater value and appeal to older adults. Communities may develop such concepts as targeted nutrition/exercise centres. Government is working to develop better guidelines and programmes for nutrition, perhaps even specialised recommendations for the physically active and the sedentary. The ideas to help us enjoy greater health-spans are countless, and their benefits will surely grow with the aging population.

ELDERLY AND PHYSICAL ACTIVITY

Increased physical activity in the elderly has been shown to increase life expectancy even into advanced old age. Many of the so-called normative changes associated with aging are not inevitable. Changes in muscle mass trigger almost all of the other changes. Studies reflect changes in almost every organ system and the skeleton. All of these changes with decreased activity reflect almost precisely the kinds of very slow changes we see with advancing age.

When athletes aged 45 to 60 were compared with athletes in their 20s, as well as inactive men in both age groups, researchers found that loss of muscle and increase fat were not age-related. The amount of fat they have stored is directly related to the amount of time they spend exercising. Related research has shown aerobic exercise causes adaptations in skeletal muscle that result in substantial increases in oxidative capacity, glycogen stores, insulin sensitivity and functional capacity in the elderly.

The most dramatic research by Evans has shown successful strength-training with the very frail elderly in nursing homes. The average age in one pilot study was 90.2 years old. Many required assistance in their daily tasks and 80 per cent had a history of falling. For eight weeks of strength training, the group lifted weights at 80 per cent of their one-repetition maximum. By the end, they increased muscle strength by 160 per cent and muscle mass by over 10 per cent. In this population, muscle is quite responsive and, in fact, it appears just as responsive to training as muscle of younger people.

Healthy aging and independent living depend upon physical activity. What types of activities interest you? Choose something that you want to do. Start slowly and build-up gradually until you are able to do 30 to 60 minutes of moderate activity most days of the week. And remember, choose activities that will:

a) build your endurance;
b) increase your flexibility; and
c) improve your strength and balance.

Physical activity is one of the most important things you can do to maintain your physical and mental health and quality of life as you get older. Walking, stretching, and keeping your muscles in good condition will help you to maintain your independence.

Physical inactivity makes your body age faster. Independent living depends on being able to do the things you want to do when you want to do them. To stay independent you need to be able to reach, bend, lift, carry, and move around easily. Staying physically active will help you to keep moving, and stay strong.

Think about the following facts:

a) 60 per cent of older adults are inactive.
b) Sitting or lying for long periods is a serious health risk.
c) Inactivity leads to declines in:
d) Bone strength;
e) Muscle strength;
f) Heart and lung fitness, and
g) Flexibility.
h) Inactivity is as harmful to your health as smoking.

Get active your way

a) at home
b) in your community
c) with friends

d) on the way to and from activities
e) Walk wherever and whenever you can.
f) Start slowly with easy stretching.
g) Move around frequently.
h) Take the stairs instead of the elevator.
i) Carry home the groceries.
j) Find activities that you enjoy.
k) Try out a class in your community.

Benefits from regular physical activity include:

a) Continued independent living
b) Better physical and mental health
c) Improved quality of life
d) More energy
e) Move with fewer aches and pains
f) Better posture and balance
g) Improved self-esteem
h) Weight maintenance
i) Stronger muscles and bones
j) Relaxation and reduced stress

Scientists have proved that being active reduces the risk of:

a) Heart disease
b) Falls and injuries
c) Obesity
d) High blood pressure
e) Adult-onset diabetes
f) Osteoporosis
g) Stroke
h) Depression

i) Colon cancer

j) Premature death.

Being active is very safe for most people. Start a physical activity programme slowly and build up. Accumulate 30 to 60 minutes of moderate physical activity most days. Minutes count—add it up 10 minutes at a time. Consult with a health-care professional.

Physical inactivity has been established as a major risk factor for the development of coronary artery disease. It also contributes to other risk factors including obesity, high blood pressure and a low level of HDL cholesterol. Even modest levels of physical activity are beneficial. Older adults and people with disabilities can gain significant health benefits with a moderate amount of physical activity, preferably daily. Physical activity need not be strenuous to bring health benefits. What is important is to include activity as part of the regular routine.

For older adults, this moderate amount of activity can come from longer sessions of moderately intense activities such as walking or swimming or shorter sessions of more vigorous activities such as fast walking or stair-climbing. Greater amounts of physical activity can bring additional benefits. But it should not be done excessively, or injury may result. People with disabilities are less likely than people without disabilities to engage in regular moderate physical activity, but they can still benefit from exercise.

Those who are physically active longer or more intensely will derive greater benefits. Scientific evidence also supports the notion that even low-intensity activities, when performed daily, can have some long-term health benefits. They help lower the risk of cardiovascular disease.

For the elderly, walking, gardening and yard work are the most popular moderate-intensity leisure activities. Golf, badminton, croquet, shuffleboard, lawn bowling and table tennis are also recommended for older people. Muscle-strengthening activities are also important for older people to reduce the risk of failing and improve the ability to perform daily tasks. The loss of strength and stamina attributed to aging is due, in part, to reduced physical activity. Both older adults and people with disabilities should consult their physicians before starting a new physical activity.

REFERENCES

Bud Getchell Alan E. Mikesky Kay Mikesky, *Physical Fitness: A Way of Life*, 1998.

Carrier, K., M. Steinhardt, and S. Bowman, 'Rethinking traditional weight management programs: A 3-year follow-up evaluation of a new approach', *Journal of Psychology* 128: 517535, 1994.

Daniel Girdano, Dorothy E. Dusek George S. Everly, *Controlling Stress and Tension*, 2001.

Darden, Ellington, *Living Longer Stronger*, New York: Burkley Publishing, 1995.

David K. Miller T. Earl Allen, *Fitness: A Lifetime Commitment*, 1995.

F.J. McGuigan, *Encyclopedia of Stress,* 1999.

Fletcher, Anne, *Thin for Life*, Shelburne, VT: Chapters Publishing, 1994.

James F. McKenzie Jan L. Smeltzer, *Planning, Implementing, and Evaluating Health Promotion Programs: A Primer*, 2001.

James J. Neutens Laurna Rubinson, *Research Techniques for the Health Sciences*, 1997

Jan Galen Bishop *Fitness Through Aerobics,* 1999.

John A. Romas M.P.H., Ph.D. Manoj Sharma M.B.B.S., Ph.D., *Practical Stress Management: A Comprehensive Workbook for Managing Change and Promoting Health*, 2000.

Joseph W. Donnelly Norm Eburne Mark Kittleson, *Mental Health: Dimensions of Self-Esteem and Emotional Well-Being*, 2001.

Kingsbury, B., *Full Figure Fitness: A Program for Teaching Overweight Adults*, Champaign, IL: Life Enhancement Publications, 1993.

Kirkley, George and John Goodbody, *The Manual of Weight Training*, London: Stanley Paul, 1994.

Larry Brown, H., *Lifetime Fitness*, 1996.

Noril, Christopher, *The Weight Training Principles and Practice Manual*, London: A & C Publishing, 1993.

Obvious Guide To Medical Survival, Thomas, Frank M., Jr. Paperback ISBN: 0970632606.

Occupational Disease in Relation to Compensation and Health Insurance (Columbia University, Studies in the Social Sciences, No 345), Goldberg, Rosamond W. Hardcover ISBN: 040451345X.

Patricia A. Reagan Jodi Brookins Fisher, *Community Health in the 21st Century*, 1997.

Rebecca J. Donatelle Lorraine G. Davis, *Access to Health*, 2000.

Scharzenegger, Arnold, *The Encyclopedia of Modern Bodybuilding*, New York: Simon and Schuster, 1987.

6

Physical Exercises for Older People

Many age-associated declines occur not because of the aging process itself, but as a result of our lifestyle habits, including exercise. In our sedentary society, many muscle and joint problems are the result of weakness and inflexibility. By increasing your strength and flexibility, you can prevent injury and slow the age-associated loss of muscle function. Inactive people become more frail than active people and are more likely to sustain a serious fall that could lead to hospitalisation, permanent disability, dependence and even death.

Exercise can slow and even reverse many components of the aging process. Proper exercise can rejuvenate you and take years off your chronological age—it is the closest thing to an anti-aging pill. In other words, exercise can add years to your life and life to your years.

Person over the age of fifty have marked increases in their muscle tone, strength and aerobic capacity: they have become more fit and vigorous then ever before. One of the things that happens when you begin strength training is that connective tissue, such as ligaments and tendons, gets stronger along with your muscles. This helps to protect your joints from injury and makes everyday tasks easier, such as walking up stairs, carrying groceries and keeping up with grandchildren.

Many wellness programmes include low-impact aerobics and strength training. Bowling, and croquet leagues are also a fun way to stay in shape. Whatever form of exercises you choose to do, you should include ones that employ a mixture of endurance, strength, balance and flexibility exercises. Before starting, check with your doctor to see if there are any medical concerns. Appropriate exercise can reduce frailty in old age thus helping to make a person's last few years be filled with active participation instead of the bedridden existence.

HOW TO REDUCE ABDOMINAL MUSCLES

The abdominals are one of the body's most talked about muscle groups. It seems like just about everyone would like to tone and/or reduce this area. Unfortunately, it is also the muscle group that generates the most misconceptions. You cannot spot reduce fat. Exercises will tone your abdominal muscles, but you will have the same layer of fat sitting on these muscles unless you create a calorie deficit by burning more calories than you consume. The most effective combination is eating low-fat foods, aerobic exercise, and strength training. You might not like this answer, but it is the only one that will work in the long run.

Many people are on a quest to achieve a 'flat stomach'. Unfortunately, this is not physiologically possible. The obsession with the abdominal area can cause frustration, anxiety, and can even lead to eating disorders. The truth is, our abdominals are not designed to be flat. Instead, the abdominal muscles form a rounded shape. The torso is shaped like a cylinder, not a laundry aid. Gender, age, and individual body types can effect the size and shape of your abdomen. So instead of worrying about something you cannot change, try focusing on something you can—like your posture. Good posture consists of a slight bending of the knees, using the abdominal muscles to point the tailbone toward the floor, and keeping your shoulders back and your head balanced on your neck. Think of a string attached to your head which is being pulled upward. Better posture will make you feel taller and slimmer.

Many people believe that performing lots of abdominal exercises is a way of achieving a flat stomach. The abdominal muscles react to resistance training just like any other muscle group. Performing 100 biceps curls is not the proper way to overload the biceps—neither is doing 100 crunches to work the abdominals. Unfortunately, many of these exercise devices that claim to trim, flatten and tone the stomach are ineffective and some are actually unsafe. You can achieve results without any equipment. You can even tone your abdominals by performing a pelvic tilt while sitting in a chair. This method can strengthen your abdominals for better posture and for supporting the back.

Fat supplies a relatively large percentage of the energy requirements during prolonged low-intensity exercise. But at this low intensity, fat is burned at a relatively slow rate. By contrast, higher-intensity aerobic exercise uses a smaller percentage of fat but results in a greater total calorie expenditure. When total fat use is calculated, researchers have found that more total fat is burned at higher exercise intensities, at least up to the highest intensity an exerciser can sustain without going to exhaustion. The selective use of fat as a fuel, specifically at lower intensities, does not translate into greater fat loss, regardless of how tempting it is to draw this conclusion.

For those who have been sedentary, high-intensity exercise compromises the ability to sustain exercise for a long time. For that reason, lower-intensity exercise is more effective in the initial stages of training and is a prerequisite to higher calorie-burning intensities. In addition, older, sedentary individuals tend to rely more on carbohydrate utilisation than do younger individuals. This does not imply that older people cannot lose fat weight as a result of training. It does mean they may need to exercise at a lower relative intensity to keep going longer, thus enhancing duration and total calorie expenditure.

Exercise fuel utilisation and post-exercise energy expenditure should not be primary considerations in fat weight control. The total amount of fat used, not the percentage of calories contributed by fat, is most important. Total calorie expenditure during exercise ultimately determines the amount of fat used.

The primary reason to use the aerobic energy system is to avoid fatigue so the exercise session can be sustained as long as possible. Using intervals potentially enables an exerciser to burn more total calories in a given session.

Because of the individual nature of exercise metabolism and the many factors involved, no single exercise/weight control prescription is ideal for everyone.

Some guidelines for becoming a calorie-burning machine are given below:

a) Develop a reasonable level of cardiorespiratory fitness.

b) To increase the rate of fat loss, gradually increase exercise duration to 50 to 60-plus minutes at least three to five days per week and raise the intensity as high as you can safely sustain it.

c) Try to include strength training twice a week to increase muscle mass.

d) Allow at least six months to realise most physiological changes and an additional six to nine months for final adaptive changes in body composition.

PROBLEMS RELATED TO SWEATING

When engaged in physical activity, body temperature rises as much as three degrees. Your body's natural cooling system, sweating, kicks in to lower body temperature. Under extreme exercise and heat stress, a body can lose 1/2 a gallon of water per hour. If the lost water is not replaced, dehydration occurs and serious consequences may follow. To understand what happens, here presented the analogy of your car. When your car's cooling system is running smoothly, excess heat from the engine is transferred to the water in the tubes, which goes to the radiator to be cooled by the air. The cooled water goes back to be heated once again by heat drawn from the engine. If there is not enough water in the system to allow for proper heat dissipation, your engine overheats, your car stops running, and you are left cursing at the side of the road. Now picture your body as the car—your muscles are the engine, your skin is the radiator and your blood vessels are the water tubes that connect the engine with the radiator. When your cooling system is running smoothly, excess heat from your muscles is drawn into your blood vessels where is circulates to your skin. Evaporating sweat draws heat away from the blood vessels. The cooler blood then recirculates throughout the body, lowering body temperature.

When too much water is lost through sweating, your blood volume decreases. This decreases blood pressure which, in turn, reduces blood flow between the muscles and skin. To overcome this, your heart rate increases. Because less blood reaches the skin, heat loss is reduced and the body overheats. If you fail to replace the water you lose, you run the risk of becoming dehydrated. When a person is dehydrated by more that four per cent or five per cent of body weight, their exercise performance declines by 20 per cent to 30 per cent. Not only that, the impact of dehydration on the cardiovascular system can produce heart problems in people with coronary heart disease and diabetes.

Sweating is not the only way you lose water. Another is through respiration—you lose water every time you exhale. This water loss increases as your physical activity increases because you breathe more. So if you are just replacing how much you are sweating out, it is not enough. If you just drink when you are thirsty, you are not getting enough water because thirst alone is not the best measure of a body is fluid needs. Generally speaking, you should drink water before, during, and after exercise. Drinking about two cups (16-oz.) of water one hour before, and one cup 1/2 hour before is a good start. Then you should drink 1/2 cup to 1 cup or more, every 15-20 min. The amount depends on the air temperature, your body weight and how hard you are exercising.

EXERCISE TO DIABETIC PERSONS

Diabetes mellitus is a condition where the body has trouble taking glucose from the blood and delivering it to the rest of the body so that it can be used as energy. This is because of a lack of, or an inability to use insulin, the hormone required to escort glucose from the blood to cells of the body. There are two common types of diabetes:

a) *Insulin-dependent diabetes mellitus (Type I)*: People who have this cannot produce insulin and must take insulin by injection. Because the medical concerns and complications, exercise for the Type I diabetic should be medically supervised.

b) *Noninsulin-dependent diabetes mellitus (Type II)*: These people are insulin resistant, meaning that they produce insulin, but it is not effective in escorting the glucose into the cells. Eighty to ninety percent of the diabetic population is Type II. A physician will prescribe oral hypoglycemic agents if blood glucose levels cannot be controlled. As a last resort, a Type II diabetic will be put on insulin, which is likely if they continue with poor lifestyle choices such as sedentary living, poor eating habits and weight gain.

Exercise has the potential to control the diabetes by nonmedical means, reduce the severity of the disease, and significantly reduce the risk of long-term complications. Aerobic exercise increases insulin sensitivity and, along with proper nutrition, helps restore normal glucose metabolism by decreasing body fat. Strength training also decreases body fat by raising the metabolism. It is main benefit, however, is increasing glucose uptake by the muscles and enhancing the ability to store glucose.

Anyone with diabetes have a thorough medical exam to see if there are risks for coronary artery disease and that blood glucose control is adequate before starting an exercise programme. The doctor will usually advise exercise if the patient has:

a) blood glucose less than 250 mg/dl.
b) no symptoms of retinopathy, neuropathy or nephropathy.
c) no cardiovascular problems such as angina, embolism, or aneurysm
d) no other condition that makes exercise inadvisable.

For a person with diabetes an open sore can turn into a serious infection so proper footwear is a must. Shoes should be comfortable, well-fitting and appropriate for the chosen exercise. Before putting on the shoes, check for pebbles or other small objects inside. Smooth, not nubby socks should be worn during exercise and changed after a workout. Sweaty socks increase the chance of getting athlete's foot. Feet are to be checked daily for scratches, cuts, blisters, ingrown toenails, corns, and calluses.

Hypoglycemia is a major risk among Type II diabetics on oral medication because of insulin-like effect of exercise. The increased glucose uptake by the muscles produces low blood glucose levels which can continue for 12-24 hours. The warning signs for mild and moderate hypoglycemic reactions are: trembling or shakiness, rapid heart rate, palpitations, increased sweating, excessive hunger, headache, drowsiness, mental confusion, and abrupt mood changes.

In the event of a hypoglycemic attack:

a) take action even if you are not sure you have hypoglycemia—waiting can make your symptoms much worse.
b) take a blood-glucose test to confirm the problem.
c) eat or drink foods with sugar such as 1/2 cup of fruit juice, six life-savers, one small box of raisins, or three glucose tablets. Food with fat should be avoided because it blocks the absorption of sugar into the bloodstream.

d) take at least a 10-15 minute rest and retest blood-glucose level before resuming exercise. Do not exercise if it is below 100 mg/dl or you still do not feel right.

e) If you do continue to exercise, be on the lookout for any signs that the hypoglycemic reaction is not over. Take your blood-glucose level at least every 20-30 minutes during your workout.

f) After your workout eat a complex carbohydrate snack.

Insulin sensitivity can remain high for 24-48 hours after a person stops exercising. Late-onset hypoglycemia is believed to be more common than hypoglycemia that occurs during or right after exercise. It is more common among new exercisers or people who exercise strenuously. You can help prevent late-onset hypoglycemia by asking your doctor about adjusting your insulin or oral medication before exercise and increasing your food intake before and after exercise.

Let your body get used to exercising. Start out easy and gradually increase intensity and duration. Warm up and cool down for 5-10 minutes each by exercising at a low intensity before and after your moderate intensity workout. Sufficient warm up and cool down will help to prevent heart problems as well as make you less susceptible to injury.

Do not exercise outdoors on very hot or humid days. You can get heat exhaustion or heat stroke. In warm weather, dress in lightweight, light-coloured, loose-fitting cotton clothing or special fabrics that promote heat loss. Wear a hat and apply sunscreen. To prevent dehydration, drink a cup of cold water before and after you exercise. If you exercise longer than 30 minutes or are sweating a lot, drink water during your workout.

Since many Type II diabetics are sedentary and overweight, low-impact exercise such as walking or stationary cycling is recommended, along with enough exercise to promote weight management. Their goal should be to exercise five times per week, up to 40-60 minutes per session at a moderate intensity. This level of exercise can be reached gradually, starting as low as 10-20 minutes a few times a week for a person who has never exercised.

For those who have no other complications, strength training is safe and can provide many benefits. It can increase lean mass which will help in weight management, as well as increase glucose uptake by the muscles and help the body to store glucose. Strength training programmes are designed around a persons needs, desires, level of conditioning and time factors. A basic recommendation from the American College of Sports Medicine is to train a minimum of two times per week, doing 8-12 repetitions per set of 8-10 exercises targeting major muscle groups. Safety precautions must be followed for the exercising diabetic. A personal trainer can help to set up a programme for the Type II diabetic and help them to exercise correctly.

Exercise and good nutrition provide real physical pay-offs—they are essential to controlling diabetes. Exercise can help prolong your life and improve the quality of your added months and years. Sticking to an exercise programme can be a challenge for anyone, even with strong medical reasons to exercise. Measuring your blood-glucose level before and after exercise can be a motivator. Diabetics who play the numbers game commonly see a twenty percent decrease in their blood-glucose level after exercising. It is crucial that the exercise be fun and there is some variety. Family support and exercising with someone are helpful.

STRENGTH TRAINING PROGRAMME

Inactive adults lose around one-half pound of muscle per year, or five pounds per decade. If you take in more calories then you burn, the extra calories get stored as fat. Fat is less dense then muscle—a pound of fat takes up more room than a pound of muscle. You need to increase your resting metabolic rate (RMR), which is the pace your body burns calories at rest. Your RMR is closely linked to the amount of muscle you have muscle burns more calories than fat. Adding muscle will raise your RMR and will greatly increase the chance that the weight loss will be maintained.

Strength training is as important, maybe more important to successful fat loss than aerobic exercise. The reason lies in the amount of calories that are burned when you are not exercising. Depending on the intensity and your weight, an aerobic workout (walking, cycling, stair-stepping) will burn approximately 300 calories per hour. If the exercise is strenuous enough (which is unlikely in the beginning exerciser) the RMR will be elevated temporarily up to a few hours afterwards. Compare this to strength training which elevates the RMR permanently.

A three-month basic strength-training programme resulted in the subjects gaining three pound of muscle and losing four pounds of fat, while eating 370 more calories per day (a 15 percent calorie increase). Remember, aerobic exercise generally does not increase muscle tissue. In fact, excessive amount of aerobic exercise combined with a low-calorie diet can cause the loss of some muscle tissue. This is not to say that overweight individuals should not do aerobic exercise—it offers many health benefits and is a part of a weight loss programme. Do not think that you need to workout in a gym for two hours to strength train. Significant gains can be made with a consistent 30-minute workout performed two/three times per week.

As we grow older we get much weaker and suffer more aches and pains. We have been told that losing muscle and gaining fat are just part of the natural aging process. The fact is that many of the symptoms of old age are really the symptoms of inactivity—of using our muscles less. Muscle weakness, bone loss, and sluggish metabolism are changes that accompany aging but are not solely caused by it.

Strength training is a potent age eraser. It is their weapon of choice for fighting physical declines associated with aging. More and more fitness experts are recommending strength training for health reasons—for women as well as men, older adults as well as younger adults. Strength training is extremely important in combating the age-related declines in muscle mass, bone density and metabolism. It is an effective way to increase muscle strength and to shed unwanted inches.

Physical inactivity causes an average muscle loss of five/seven pounds per decade. This muscle loss leads to a metabolic rate reduction of two/five per cent per decade. Calories that were previously used for muscle energy are put into fat storage, resulting in gradual weight gain. One study on older adults showed that a three month basic strength-training programme resulted in the exercisers adding three pounds of muscle and losing four pounds of fat, while eating 15 more calories.

Sensible strength training may be one of the best ways to get relief from your arthritis. Not only will it help to lubricate and nourish the joint, strength training will also strengthen the muscles around the joint, providing it with greater support. Strength training can add bone density.

The Simple Fitness Solutions Strength-Training Kit is perfect for the person over fifty who wants a simple, safe, effective, and inexpensive way to train at home. It includes a set of two rubber tubing rings with foam handles and a training booklet that describes a strength training and flexibility routine that will work all the major muscle groups in only 30 minutes. The exercises are easy to follow with simple language and line drawings. Rubber tubing is an effective tool for strength training. When you strength train, your muscles exert a force against some type of resistance.

Home-based resistance training programme utilising elastic tubing can serve as a practical, effective means of eliciting strength gains in adults over the age of 65. Elastic tubing is inexpensive, compact and easy to use, and is therefore a convenient means of strength training for those who are older and on limited incomes. As you get stronger with strength training, you will need added resistance in order to improve. If you are using dumbbells, you need to use heavier weights—this can get costly and cumbersome. With rubber tubing, you simply move it farther to make an exercise harder. Also, rubber tubing will allow you to train muscles that dumbbells can not train in a seated position, such as the chest and mid-back.

The strength-training kit is safe, effective, time efficient, easy to follow, economical and reliable. The training booklet contains exercises that are illustrated and written in simple language. It also contains guidelines on proper form, posture and safe techniques, as well as tips for sticking with your programme, a chart for logging your training, and stretches to do after your training session.

Strength training can improve the quality of your life at any age or condition. Traditionally it was thought that it was normal to get weak and feeble as one aged. You can maintain your independence and mobility far beyond your expectations as you age by simply doing strength training for 30 minutes, twice a week.

REFERENCES

David K. Miller T. Earl Allen, *Fitness: A Lifetime Commitment*, 1995.

Hoeger, Werner and Sharon Hoeger, *Lifetime Physical Fitness And Wellness*, Englewood, CO: Morton Publishing, 1992.

Larry Brown, H., *Lifetime Fitness*, 1996.

McGuigan, F.J., *Encyclopedia of Stress,* 1999.

Jan Galen Bishop *Fitness Through Aerobics,* 1999.

On The Run: Exercise And Fitness For Busy People, Waitz, Grete Paperback ISBN: 1579542530.

Weider, Joe and Bill Reynolds, *Ultimate Bodybuilding*, Chicago: Contemporary Books, 1989.

7

Essence of Yoga

With the increasing advances in medicine, it is possible to treat and control most diseases. But the side effects of every kind of medication are to be reckoned with. To carry on the analogy of a machine, proper maintenance of our body keeps it going without problems to a ripe old age. The practice of yogic asanas and pranayama is unquestionably an ideal method to preserve the health and longevity of our body.

Yoga is unique in that it recuperates the system. Due to internal massage, the cells are made to liberate their toxins more efficiently. Blood flow is increased with augmented oxygen delivery to the tissues. The question of exercise-induced free radicals never arises with the yogic system. With the mind controlling the functions of the body in the practice of yoga, cellular malfunction is prevented. The mind is kept in contact with the cells and action is based on the input from the periphery. The adjustment is deliberate, and the practitioner's awareness is so refined that he becomes conscious of the subtle functioning or malfunctioning of any part of the body. There is enough time to impose corrective action, as the practice is slow and steady.

Asanas work on gross and micro structures. The effects on cartilage, synovial lining and bone can be directly observed as asanas are practised. As the actions in asanas are both contractions and extensions, both the softness and rigidity of connective tissue are preserved. Due to the peculiar nature of yogic movements, the body is shaped and sculpted so that fat formation is optimum, and a person never gains or loses more than what is needed in the relevant areas.

Yoga is a conscious, yet an automatic, massage process in a geometric manner without actually touching the tissue with the hands. Yoga acts on the joints unlike any other system. The joints are given an internal massage. The internal tissues are aligned and massaged in an anatomical manner. This is known as servicing the joint. Smooth, soft, supple movements with alignment, and a steady state of stretch or contraction, are available only in yoga. The range of movements far surpasses that in any other science. This ensures that the joint is used through the full range of movement. While practising yoga, the mind is trained to be aware of multiple joints for alignment and other minute details.

To maintain life in any part stretching is important. Cells that are subjected to stretching are able to grow better, adapt and survive. Yogis are said to have had long lives; this was because of the kind of exercise they did on a long-term basis. Yoga does not allow bulging of cells. One can now see that yogis have had a better understanding of the human body. In the type of stretch or contraction given in yoga, the muscles are precisely positioned in certain planes and alignment is given before the stretch commences. The regional blood flow changes, but without any reflex change in any other parameter. As there is no repetitive movement, the muscles do not get exhausted.

In yoga, adequate time and a varied geometry are available to push the blood, with varying stresses and strains, even to the remotest of areas. In standing poses, the skin is trained to become highly sensitive as a tactile instrument. Touch, pressure, vibration, temperature and pain sensations of the body are sharpened. As the adjustment in standing poses are from segment to segment, every pore of the skin serves as an afferent instrument sending relays to the brain for efferent action of correction in posture. The sensory nerve endings on the skin are razor sharp due to the stretch given to them by the asanas.

The blood supply to skin is enhanced by the asanas, preventing senile changes in the skin. The healthy functioning of the organs of perception also depends on the nerve endings in the skin. Standing poses tone up peripheral circulation. All parts of the skin are made to open up and healthy sweating occurs. The heat developed is not excessive.

The asanas, by virtue of their different geometric shapes, stretch or contract every part of the skin. In inversions, the entire surface of the skin on the body becomes cool, which the practitioner can actually feel. In forward bends, the skin on the front of the body is contracted, with reduction in blood flow and increase in temperature. The blood flow on the posterior aspect is enhanced due to the stretch, the skin becoming warm initially and cool later on. The facial skin is particularly cooled, even during asana practice. In twistings, the skin is stretched, contracted and massaged. The effect is one of softening, better blood flow, no stagnation of secretions which can result in bacterial infections such as boils, warts and cysts.

Sweating patterns are moderate to intense. The skin on the abdominal area is always warm due to the repeated action of contraction, though it is also extended at times. If balancing poses are completed with urdhva dhanurasana, the skin on the abdominal surface is stretched and cooling occurs later on. Back bends stretch the front of the body. The skin on the posterior aspect contract and sweats due to the heat generated as the muscles contract intensely. The facial skin becomes warm due to the load on the skull and organs of perception in back bends. The skin on the posterior aspect of the legs also becomes warm due to the contraction, the front of the legs remaining cooler. In pranayama, as the entire mind and body are kept silent, the whole surface of the body is cooled.

Yoga practices are found highly beneficial for the proper functioning of various body processes. Almost all the systems of our body—circulatory system, respiratory system, digestive system, immune system, nervous system—are get benefited from yoga practices.

A healthy cardiovascular system prevents many other disorders as all systems are interrelated. The massaging action of asanas is valuable for the interstitial space, which improves micronutrition by healthy lymphatic flow. Arteries and veins are massaged and kept elastic, and atherosclerotic blockages prevented. The heart and the arteries remain soft and supple with the capacity to adapt. This means that even under conditions of stress, the system does not malfunction. This is real inner strength. Yoga is the only means to provide this as cellular mechanisms are regulated in the yogic system.

Yoga has provided the science of pranayama to preserve the respiratory system. Pranayama strengthens the inner vital energy at microcellular levels. This vital body cannot be measured by any medical means and is the very source of energy within us. It is essential to retain the elasticity of the lungs, to increase the uptake of oxygen, ventilate every cell in the lungs, and massage the lungs to promote longevity. Yoga ideally suits this need.

Asanas promote and maintain the elasticity of the ribs and intercostal muscles. The diaphragm is also attended to by all asanas working in different directions. Standing poses stimulate the lung. Inverted poses, by virtue of the weight of the abdominal organs on the diaphragm, toughen the lungs. Forward bends train one to breathe in a limited cavity. Twisting poses work on the same principle, but in an asymmetrical manner. Back bends are ideal for invigoration, promote excellent immunity, strengthen blood circulation in the entire lower respiratory tract.

Pranayama maintains cellular integrity of the respiratory passages excellently. The cartilages of the trachea and smaller bronchi are toned up by asanas and pranayama. They remain soft and elastic. The vocal cords are kept resilient by pranayama, and inverted asanas improve blood supply to the same area.

Asanas can massage the gastrointestinal tract. They promote expulsion of excessive wind; maintain perisitic functions, blood supply, and freshness of the tissues; and regulate transit time. The esophagus and stomach are benefited by all asanas, particularly back bends. Motility and blood supply are increased and all physiological functions toned up. The pancreas is benefited by rotational movements as it lies perpendicular to the axis of the spine. Inverted twisting poses like parivrittaikapada, sirsasana are very helpful. Back bends, are valuable to improve blood supply to the organ and freshen the cells.

A healthy flow of blood brings in its wake immune cells to circulate properly in the substance of the liver. Twisting poses are invaluable for all liver disorders as are back bending poses. If the contractions of the gall bladder are not healthy, stagnation can predispose the organ to stones. Asanas massage the gall bladder and prevent any stagnation of secretions. They keep the lining of the gall bladder healthy and ensure proper peristaltic contractions in response to hormones.

The kidney is a vital organ performing many functions. Many die from renal disease due to different causes. Diabetic renal disease is particularly disabling. The tissues are damaged by deposits of excessive cellular matrix. The increased sugar alters the structure of peptides. The arteries become thick. Asanas can prevent these changes, provided the diabetic starts yoga at an early stage. Asanas massage the kidneys and prevent degenerative changes. Back bends are valuable for this purpose. Ascending infection from the bladder can be prevented by regular practice of inverted asanas. Baddha konasana is invaluable for preventing inflammation of the urethra in both males and females. Recurrent urethritis can be prevented by these asanas.

Asanas massage the tissues and preserve a fluid state of circulation. In yoga, the auto massage on the tissues breaks any plaque that forms on the vessel wall. Anti-clotting factors are mobilised, with endocrine alterations. The massaging action of asanas brings the muscles closer to the bone, pushing blood into the marrow which is responsible for healthy cell production.

The increase in immunity levels of the body in yogic practice is due to the reduction of stress levels of the mind and body, and pooling of blood in the different parts of the body.

As the asana is discontinued slowly, the pooled blood remains in that area for some time. As such stimuli are applied daily, the body remains healthy and is never prone to infection. Again, the massage to the bone results in healthy production of blood cells. The massage to the spleen, thymus, and the circulatory system, including the lymphatics and the nodes, results in an alert and energised immune system. No stagnation of bacterial debris is allowed and disposal of waste material is efficient. Massage of the tissues and bringing forward the immune cells to remain in the area is an important mechanism in yoga.

Our system functions in an orderly manner only when there is a certain amount of quietitude. In such situations no disorderly functioning of immune cells can happen, as in autoimmune dysfunction. The massage to the skin increases blood flow to those areas which enhance and maintain healthy output of antibacterial secretions to promote immunity. The blood circulation to the lack sebaceous glands, is promoted by asanas and this develops local immunity. Mucociliary clearance systems are stimulated, aiding the immune system to function better.

The main aim of asanas is to preserve glandular function and maintain energy. The stimulation does not exhaust glandular secretions. Hence, the practitioner emerges fresh even after two hours of yoga—actually fresher than prepractice levels. Power and vitality are side effects of good glandular function. All asanas are useful, particularly inverted poses. Back bends stimulate, forward bends recuperate, passive poses energise the system. Asanas have stimulating and suppressive effects on the male sexual organs. Forward bends, baddha konasana, upavishta and samakonasana inhibit physical stimulation. Back bends increase the strength of the sexual drive and the contracting capacity of the muscles of ejection.

Pranayama, by its dissociation of the mind from the senses, controls mental drive over the physical organs.

The concept of the nervous system in yogic thought is most interesting. According to Western medicine, there are several major and sub-plexuses along the entire length of the body in front of the vertebral column. Some of the major ones are the coccygeal plexus, sacral plexus, lumbar plexus, hypogastric plexus, coeliac plexus, epigastric or solar plexus, gastric plexus, cardiac plexus, cervical plexus, and pharyngeal plexus. All are in communication with each other, and with the sympathetic and parasympathetic nervous systems.

Yogic texts describe centres or chakras which are points of energy. These are not physical matter but energy centres. Mastery of the functioning of each of these leads to specific capabilities. According to yogic texts, two types of energy, positive and negative, represented by the pingala and the ida nerves, pervade the body. The pingala is on the right side of the body and the ida on the left. The pingala stimulates the functions of the mind and body, while the ida suppresses them. This aptly corresponds to the sympathetic and parasympathetic nervous systems.

The human body can be described as being made up of three parts: the *sthula sharira* or gross body; the *karana sharira* or causal body; and the *sukshma sharira* or subtle body. The yogic chakras and nerve plexuses that correspond with each other are described below:

a) *Muladhara chakra*: The muladhara chakra is situated in the pelvis. The chakra is concerned with nourishment, absorption and elimination of waste matter. It is the seat of the annamaya kosa or the body of nourishment. Mastery of this chakra also leads to control of sexual energy. According to medicine, the inferior hypogastric plexus innervates the organs of the pelvic cavity and muscles of the rectum, with fibres to the penis and sensory fibres to the vagina. It is joined by branches from the 2nd, 3rd and

4th sacral nerves. The pelvic organs are actually supplied by the pelvic plexus which is a branch of the hypogastric plexus.

A part of the large intestine and the rectum are supplied by nerves from the superior hypogastric plexus which has communication with the sympathetic and parasympathetic nerve, the vagus. The coeliac plexus is one of the largest plexuses of the autonomic system. It is situated at the level of the first lumbar vertebra. The coeliac ganglia also supplies part of the large intestine. The small intestine is concerned with absorption of food. The small intestine is supplied by the coeliac ganglia. Hence, the muladhara chakra controls the functions of these plexuses.

b) *Svadhishthana chakra*: The svadhishthana chakra, situated above the organs of generation, corresponds to and controls, part of the hypogastric plexus which supplies nerve fibres to the colon, prostate, uterus and vagina. This chakra is the element of water and smell. The colon is important for absorption of water and balance of the moisture content of the faecal matter, and hence, the tissues of the body.

c) *Manipuraka chakra*: The manipuraka chakra in the navel area is the element of fire. It controls and corresponds to the gastric plexus which supplies the stomach and, in conjunction with the vagus, controls acid flow in the organ.

d) *Surya chakra*: The surya chakra corresponds to the solar or epigastric plexus which lies behind the stomach and innervates all the abdominal organs. From the epigastric plexus are derived all the plexuses: the renal, suprarenal, spermatic, coeliac, superior mesentric and aortic plexuses. The coeliac plexus of nerves forms the coeliac ganglia and gives rise to the phrenic, gastric, hepatic and splenic plexuses.

e) *Manas chakra*: The manas chakra lies between the surya and the anahata chakras. It is the seat of emotion, imagination and creativity.

f) *Anahata chakra*: The anahata chakra lies in the region of the physical heart. It corresponds to the cardiac plexus.

g) *Visuddhi chakra*: The visuddhi chakra lies in the region of the throat, above the chest at the base of the neck, and corresponds to the cervical and pharyngeal plexus. It represents the intellectual sheath—the vijnanamaya kosa.

h) *Ajna chakra*: The ajna chakra represents the abode of joy—anandamaya kosa and lies in the centre of the forehead. This corresponds to the region of the thalamus. When activated, the person is always joyful. It actually means that equanimity is mastered and the person is naturally blissful.

i) *Lalata chakra*: The lalata chakra is at the top of the forehead, corresponding to the cortical centres. It helps proper awareness and perfect action in all situations.

j) *Soma chakra*: Soma chakra cools the body, akin to that part of the hypothalamus which has receptors for regulation of body temperature.

k) *Sahasrara chakra*: Sahasrara chakra is the centre of the supreme spirit. Mastery of this means liberation. This is the harmonious functioning of all parts of the mind and brain, thus qualifying for the state of samadhi.

Nadies are channels for passage of vital energy. The nadis penetrate the entire body from the soles to the crown of the head. All nadis originate from the kandasthana and the heart. Twelve digits above the anus, and just below the navel, is a bulb known as the kanda. This releases 72,000 nerves, and from each of them another 72,000 branch off.

According to *Shiva Samhita* there are 350,000 nadis. The three most important are the ida, pingala and susumna. The susumna lies in the centre of the spinal column and this position corresponds to the central nervous system of modern anatomy. The ida starts in the left nostril, goes to the crown of the head and then downwards to the base of the spine. The pingala nadi does likewise, starting from the right nostril. Solar energy is said to flow through it, hence it is also called the surya nadi. The ida is the chandra nadi, or the conduit for lunar energy. The ida and pingala nerves criss-cross at the chakras, and are, therefore, interconnected with the susumna. This is also true of Western thought where it is said that the sympathetic and parasympathetic nerves are in connection with the nerve plexuses and with the spinal cord.

The other important nadis are: gandhari, originating in the left eye; hastijihva, in the right eye; pusa, in the right ear; yasasvini, in the left ear; alambusa, in the mouth; kuhu, in the genital region; sankhini, in the anus. Nadis may also correspond to arteries, veins, and the channels and ducts of all the systems. They function as inlets and outlets of various energies.

According to the *Shiva Samhita*, when food is digested, nadis take the best part of the nourishment to the subtle body (*sukshma sharira*), the middle part to the gross body (*sthula sharira*), and the inferior part is discharged as faeces, urine and sweat. Nadikas are smaller nadis and nadi chakras are ganglia. Modern science has also described nerves for every part of the body, but the difference, according to yogic thought, is that these nerves cannot function by themselves but have vital airs that enable them to function. These airs are: *prana*, *udana*, *samana*, *vyana*, *apana*, *naga*, *kurma*, *krkara*, *devadatta* and *dhananjaya*.

a) *Prana* vitalises the heart.

b) *Udana* activates the throat (melodious voice).

c) *Samana* energises the navel region (digestion).

d) *Vyana* is crucial in the entire body.

e) *Apana* is vigorous in the region of the anus.

f) *Naga* is essential to the act of belching.

g) *Kurma* opens the eyelid.

h) *Krkara* causes sneezing.

i) *Devadatta* is responsible for yawning.

j) *Dhananjaya* pervades the entire frame, even after death.

Though modern anatomy assigns specific nerves for each part of the body, sometimes it cannot explain functional disorders. A situation often arises in clinical medicine when investigations do not reveal any abnormality even when the patient demonstrates clear symptoms. The physician is left with no method to treat such a situation. A simple example is that of a burning sensation in the stomach not related to stress or any type of food. If investigations do not reveal any pathology, the problem is labelled as a functional disorder. No remedy in Western medicine helps. In such a situation, yoga says that the gastric fire—manipuraka chakra—suffers over-stimulation. Back bends are prescribed and the patient gets the necessary relief.

Practice of yoga regulates the health of the nervous system. The chakras are activated and the practitioner remains alert to a ripe old age. All asanas are useful. Standing poses stimulate the chakras. Back bends are the ones that stimulate the chakras vigorously. Forward bends soothe chronic headaches while back bends strengthen the nerves to prevent headaches. All nerve roots are toned up by asanas. The spinal cord is massaged, and the blood supply to the cord is maintained. Inversions preserve all neurological functions of the brain. They maintain healthy electrical transmission in the brain and prevent senility. Asanas and pranayama refresh the mind as recuperation occurs. The sympathetic and parasympathetic nervous systems are the gates through which yoga works.

Practice of yoga deeply affects the special senses. Eyes are the areas where tension and fatigue show up earliest. The use of bandages over the eyes in asana and pranayama practice cuts off visual sensation. This is useful in certain cases of glaucoma, hypertension and nervous fatigue. The wetness of the tissue of the eye is preserved. The entire structure of the orbit remains soft, elastic and healthy. Formation of cataracts can be arrested to a great extent by head stand.

Auditory sensations are also toned up by yogic asanas. The blood supply to the inner ear is enhanced preventing senile nerve deafness. The integrity of the delicate balancing mechanism is preserved. Inverted asanas are valuable for this, especially sarvangasana and half halasana. Back bends maintain the vibratory capacity of the bony ossicles. This also helps prevent age-related hearing loss.

Practice of pranayama with the bandage removes stress from the eye and ear. The mind is taken deep into the consciousness and introspection occurs. The loss of contact with the external world provides rest for the eye and ear. After prolonged practice of asanas and pranayama, the taste buds become razor sharp. This is something that can only be subjectively experienced. Sitali pranayama is the only type where the tongue is opened and folded like a leaf. This invigorates the taste buds on the tongue. It also affects the flow of saliva. In fact, when one gets up from savasana after a practice of pranayama, the secretions in the mouth are virtually nil. This is a sign of temporary hibernation.

Yoga provides relaxation to the body by working through the special senses. The very perception of the relaxation is through the special senses. In this context, it is very useful to understand the value of the yogic technique called shanmukhi mudra which provides complete neuromuscular relaxation to the special senses. The electrical nerves of the eye, ear and face are relaxed in this practice, and when the nerves are relaxed, their function is razor sharp.

Methods of exercising in yoga arc different from any other exercise system. The mind is given immense importance, there are precise explanations and instructions on various aspects like timing and sequence of asanas. It is a detailed science and in order to understand it, it is important to know why we should exercise at all. Many people do not exercise and yet live to a ripe old age. But the quality of life of such persons will not be as good as one would like it to be. Yoga is the only tool that can maintain health in a cellular sense. It is non-invasive and without side effects. However, practice of asanas and pranayama needs *tapas* (motivation). This is preventive medicine according to ancient logic. To undertake preventive steps one must understand the effects of aging on the human body. Aging is the diminished ability of the cells of the body to react and adjust to the internal and external environment.

YOGA AND SPORTS

Physical activity is of extreme benefit to the body, it can produce the necessary chemical changes in the body. It is essential that the sportsperson includes recreational in daily life. Yoga is an ideal means for protecting the mind and body of the athlete. The ordinary player will find yoga useful to combat physical and mental stress brought on by the game. The professional athlete will realise it to be an invaluable means of reaching and maintaining the peak of physical and mental strength. If activities involving body movements are done without mental tension, stress relief results. However, as sport is becoming more and more professionalised, a sportsperson much greater suffer stress than, for example, an executive. The latter uses physical activity to remove physiological and psychological stress. In the case of the professional sportsperson, the right approach is to use yoga to relieve stress on the body and mind.

One main concern is that some sporting activities rely on usage of one part of the body, and this creates asymmetry and overuse of that part. All kinds of sporting activities are gaining ground—jumping from a high cliff for the thrill of it, with ropes attached to the legs, is one form of sport that can be particularly strenuous and harmful to the joints of the lower limb. Many such equally harmful activities exist and the list increases every day. When ordinary sporting events are loaded with potential harm, one can understand the dangers in the newer kinds of sporting activities.

The five basic ingradients a sportsperson needs are: speed, flexibility, endurance, strength and stamina. We would add a sixth aspect—mental fortitude along the lines of Patanjali. This is not purely a physiological phenomenon, but a complex interplay of mind and body.

Pranayama builds up endurance, courage, vital strength due to refreshment of the nervous system, and skill due to a serene mind. The vital strength of the cardiac and respiratory systems are improved by pranayama. Any sportsperson who has to move about constantly will benefit in hockey, football, basket ball, boxing, swimming, golf, cycling, skiing, rowing. In swimming, particularly, the various types of pranayama with the use of bandhas and kumbakhas are helpful in preventing exhaustion of the lungs in water. A certain quietitude is needed in some events like archery, shooting and golf. Steadiness of the nerves is essential for skill in these events, and pranayama, by quietening the organs of perception, provides a withdrawal. This stabilises and steadies the electrical function of the nerves.

The daily life of a sportsperson calls for scientific systematisation of the time of training and regularisation in intake of a balanced diet of protein, carbohydrates and fat. Depending on the type of sport, the training routine varies and the type of side effects on the body also varies.

The impact of sporting activities on the human body needs to be discussed as this is of vital importance and singnificance.

The heart of a sportsperson is larger in size than that of a normal person. This is due to the effects of training. The ventricles, on account of their bulk, need to contract only a little to push out the blood. In a normal person, a complete contraction is needed for this. Both aerobic and anaerobic capacity are greater of value in endurance events. Some studies have reported symptoms of giddiness, exhaustion and light headedness with endurance training, but this could represent a factor of overtraining. The blood is kept more fluid and fibrinolytic mechanisms are favoured, which means that the tendency for clotting is less. This is also balanced by a rise in clotting mechanisms, lest the anticlotting tide overtake the health of the body.

According to the studies in science of yoga, the sportsperson has a irritated type of circulatory status even though it may appear to function healthily. A healthy circulation is ensured by yoga as a non-irritative stimulation to the sympathetic nervous system. It leads to a restful increase in the blood flow to different parts of the body. A special problem in the athlete is orthostatic intolerance, or the inability to stand still in one place. When we stand still, the blood pools in the vessels of the legs and the volume returning to the heart is less.

In a normal person, the nervous system, in its control over the altered situation, is able to cope. In a highly trained athlete, the increase in the blood volume is several times higher than normal. This somehow alters the response of the nervous system which fails to make appropriate adjustments in the standing posture, and the athlete experiences giddiness. Such changes do not happen to the yogic practitioner. The nature of stimulus being different, a healthy resilience of circulatory flow is maintained. Even if there are problems of circulatory maladjustment with posture, asanas and pranayama can correct them by regulating the nerves which control blood pressure. Hence, an athlete would benefit by incorporating yogic practice in the daily routine.

If the intensity and duration of the exercise are increased, it becomes necessary for the body to dissipate the excess heat developed. The blood flow to the skin increases and the vessels dilate. Both these functions are controlled by the sympathetic nervous system. In severe training, the blood flow is also preferentially shunted to the vital organs, and a dual state of circulatory adjustment exists. Depending on the type of sport and the parts of the body used, the temperature of the skin rises in some areas and decreases in others.

In contrast, during yogic practice, the reflex vasodilation of the vessels is made voluntary—the practitioner has the time to adjust the geometric shape of the asana to suit the need.

Forward bends 'cool' the system and this effect can be perceived by the practitioner immediately, just as the athlete can perceive the flushing effect of the increased flow to the face during intense training.

Moreover, during asana practice, the type of stimulus used to enhance the blood flow is softer and slower, the metabolic rate of the body not being disturbed as in athletic training. The quality of blood flow as well as the effect on the skin due to habitual practice of asanas is quite different from that due to sports activities.

The skin of a sportsperson is hard and gritty, while that of the yogic practitioner is soft, supple and glossy. Alignment is also given to the skin, stretching or contracting it in a very precise manner. In sports, the nature of stimulus to the nerves that control blood flow is of high intensity and in spurts, while in asana practice the stimulus is slow and steady.

In sports training, the skin receives blood flow with a pulsatile quality due to the increased heart rate. In asana practice, the flow is slow, gentle and of a wafting quality, more conducive to cellular health in the long run. If needed, even a dynamic quality of blood flow can be imparted, especially in the practice of back bends. The generation of heat during endurance training is swift and forcible, while in yoga it is steady and controlled.

In general, the standing poses create a warm feeling in the legs due to increase in blood flow; the forward bends cool the brain and face, while heating the posterior aspect of the body. The reverse occurs in the practice of back bends. Head and shoulder stand invigorates and cools the tissues of the face. In all these poses, the blood flow to other areas is also altered if needed, depending on the type of pose.

The haematology of persons associated with endurance events may vary in comparison with those associated with power training. Red cell mass is also related to lean body mass, and to height, weight and sex. Higher counts of haemoglobin and red cell mass have been found in males due to the circulating testosterone levels. Training increases the number of white blood corpuscles in circulation and studies reveal differences in the sexes, as males generally train more intensively than females due to their greater physical capacity.

A sportsperson's aerobic capacity is far greater than that of an average lay person. As the lungs are stimulated every day by different methods, they adapt to the strain and help perform the particular sporting activity without difficulty. This is a matter of adapting and conditioning the respiratory system to the stimulus, and the training is task specific. A sprinter will not be able to do a marathon run and vice versa.

As each type of sport requires specific training, it is impossible to train the lungs for all facets of sporting activities. One has to push the system to maximum aerobic capacity to achieve proper oxygen utilisation and health of the skeletal system. This is erroneous. What is required is that the vitality of the system is retained as one grows older. This is achieved easily by the practice of asanas, where all kinds of body functions are toned up. The lungs are toned up by the practice of back bends which give an effect similar to aerobic exercises, but yet the perceived exertion is different.

The body can be toned up without the usual notion of exertion. The exertion in yoga is of a different type. The body is certainly trained to increase the intake of oxygen, but usage is curtailed at the same time, and thus the energy level is not exhausted but improved. All the parts of the body involved in oxygen transport to the cells are toned up to the maximum and the elasticity of the tissues is sustained. This maintains the delivery of the nutrients to the tissues even as a person gets older. No doubt the oxygen usage in aerobic training is higher and the body is fitter than an untrained body, but this is at the cost of many adaptive changes. In yoga, the health of the system is maintained without any change in such parameters.

Yoga is an energy-conserving exercise while sports is energy exhausting in nature. Back bends produce the effect of having run a mile race in a few minutes. The expansion of the lungs is the maximum that can ever be achieved. Forward bends train the posterior lungs, while lateral bends and rotations act on different parts of the lungs. Pranayama maximises endurance, especially if the kumbhakas are properly performed.

Prolonged exercise training actually suppresses appetite rather than increasing it, even if an acute bout of exercise increases the appetite soon after. The role of the mind is a crucial deciding factor in this. Any change in the body due to training is influenced by the mind.

The mechanical and absorptive capacities are regularised by practising yoga. Depending on the type of asana used, the entire digestive tract can be either stimulated or soothed. Nevertheless, the effect of endurance training will be neutralised by asana practice as balance of sympathetic and parasympathetic activity is obtained. If a person feels somewhat hungry before starting yoga, the hunger pangs are numbed during the practice and reappear when the practice is over. Hunger can also be reduced or enhanced by yoga, depending on the need.

The nervous system is deeply affected by yoga practice. The sympathetic tone is overcome by the parasympathetic tone with chronic training. This results in lower pulse rate and heart rate at rest. These changes revert to normalcy with deconditioning in a variable period. During exercise the athlete is able to use the sympathetic system effectively. In a normal person at rest, there is a balance between the activity of the sympathetic and parasympathetic nervous systems. Due to constant bombardment of the nerves with high intensity stimulus of an aerobic nature, the balance is reset with a predominant vagal tone.

Sports demand fast physiological responses. The mind and body are tuned to such situations. The role of the mind in improving nervous reflexes cannot be underestimated. The sympathetic and parasympathetic nervous systems balance each other during severe exercise. Noradrenaline and adrenaline are released by the nerves of the sympathetic system. These interact with alpha and beta receptors in blood vessels. Adrenaline reacts with both types and noradrenaline with only alpha receptors.

The autonomic system is balanced and quietened in the practice of asanas. Hence, the athlete would never suffer exhaustion or orthostatic intolerance. As the endogenous stimulation of the body in a person is both chemical and nervine, great energy is available to athletes who practise yoga.

Endocrine system is poised to respond very fast to challenging situations. There are a variety of adaptions that occur in the body of a trained sportsperson.

Insulin: Blood levels of glucose are initially high to meet the needs of the exercise and diminish as the body is depleted of its store. Insulin levels also fall simultaneously. This helps minimise the use of glucose by non-active tissues and spares the energy for the active muscles. In trained individuals, the level of insulin does not fall as in untrained persons.

Glucagon: Glucagon is secreted by the alpha cells of the pancreas in response to the low levels of blood glucose. It has two functions: glycogenolysis and neoglucogenesis. In prolonged exercise, the blood glucose level is maintained by this hormone in response to diminishing levels.

Catecholamines: In moderate exercise the levels of adrenaline and noradrenaline do not change, but in severe exercise the levels rise dramatically. Noradrenaline levels exceed adrenaline levels five-fold. The release of these hormones is diminished by training. Adrenaline stimulates glycogenolysis during exercise. It also stimulates lipolysis by the enzyme lipase. The blood levels of free fatty acids rise. The rise of adrenaline is greater in static exercises and of noradrenaline in dynamic types. Muscles are a major source of adrenaline during exercise. Catecholamines are released from sympathetic nerve terminals and the adrenal medulla.

Growth Hormone (GH): Growth hormone is released in response to intermittent and continuous exercise. For certain biochemical reasons, neural factors assume more importance with regard to GH during exercise. The magnitude of the response is related to the peak of exercise. The release of GH is pulsatile, so exercise once started should continue in a steady manner to ensure regular pulsatile release.

Adrenal axis: In prolonged exercise, the hypothalamus stimulates the pituitary to release the hormone ACTH. This stimulates the release of cortisol from the adrenal gland which induces proteolysis in muscles. Thus, cortisol normalises the diminishing levels of blood glucose during exercise through breakdown of amino acids.

Thyroid hormone: Hormones from the thyroid gland generally stimulate the body metabolism, rate of oxygen consumption, protein synthesis, lipolysis and glycogenolysis. The thyroid hormone acts through other hormones.

Anti-diuretic hormone (ADH): In endurance activity, it is essential that the levels of fluid and electrolytes be maintained. In response to sweating, the nuclei in the hypothalamus are stimulated, and these prompt the posterior part of the pituitary to release ADH. ADH stimulates the cells of the kidneys to retain water. If dehydration occurs, the pressure in the blood vessels falls and this again provokes ADH release to retain water and increase the blood pressure.

Yoga is useful to prevent hormonal readjustments arising out of athletic training. Asanas like head and shoulder stand, forward bends, half halasana and passive back bends soothe, refresh, and invigorate the glandular system respectively.

In human beings, the metabolic rate determines the long-term effect of endurance training. It also establishes the caloric cost of the exercise. This helps determine the nutrition needs. After maximal exercise, the oxygen consumption does not return to normal levels immediately, but in a curvilinear fashion. This extra oxygen consumption, due to the elevation of the tissue metabolic rate, has been termed the oxygen debt. During exercise, the turnover of lactic acid is several times greater than at rest. The metabolism of proteins, fats and carbohydrates depends on the hormonal responses.

Intense training can double the levels of availability of amino acids. The conversion of alanine to glucose occurs in the liver. To support prolonged exercise bouts, amino acids serve as important fuel bases. It appears that they may contribute as much as five per cent to ten per cent of the source of fuel for muscle contraction during a marathon race. It is well known that heavy exercise induces a greater loss of protein through the kidneys.

For prolonged aerobic activities, lipid is a primary source of energy. In prolonged high intensity bouts, fat is an important source of energy. The high energy content per unit weight of fat provides a vast source of potential energy reserves. But fat needs to be oxidised before use, in contrast to sugars. Endurance training improves the ability of fat usage by improving the blood flow and the mitochondrial content in skeletal muscle. In prolonged exercise, free fatty acids provide approximately 70 per cent oxidative fuel as compared to glucose.

Individuals who train substantially have lower triglycerides and higher HDL levels. Fats are used during low intensity aerobic exercise. The sparing of glycogen during endurance activities slows down the use of the same. For prolonged submaximal exercise, oxidation of fatty acids provides the maximum energy. Respiration also changes, allowing greater use of fatty acids.

Carbohydrates can be degraded without the direct use of oxygen. During prolonged exercise, glycogenolysis provides a large amount of fuel for muscle contractions. Skeletal muscle has a high glycolytic capacity. Exercising muscle may increase glucose intake eight to twenty-fold, and this is met by increased glucose production and mobilisation. To prevent hypoglycemia, free fatty acids are mobilised and utilised to the same extent as glucose during moderate exercise.

Several hormones play a role in this during severe endurance work. Catecholamines, glucagon, growth hormone and cortisol increase, while the level of insulin decreases. All these ensure hepatic output of glucose and peripheral lipid mobilisation during exercise. These neuro-endocrine changes ensure the maximum amount of energy the muscles need. Muscle biopsies done on professional athletes give evidence of the glycogen-sparing effect.

The major difference between yoga and endurance training is the method of metabolically stimulating the body. For example, forward bends reduce the metabolic rate of the body and energise the system. It is like coming out of hibernation. Back bends stimulate the body and the heat can be felt. Certain asanas warm up select areas of the body. In the forward bends, the face feels cool while the gastric area can get 'hot'. Hunger pangs are felt. The muscles of the spine on the back feel warm. In the back bends, the muscles on the front of the body feel the heat. Thus, regional control of metabolism is possible in yoga. Depending on the geometric shape of the asana, the body can either have a uniform metabolic change or different changes at different points simultaneously.

Exercise is a potent stimulator of bone formation and somehow influences remodelling. In recent years, many new facets have been discovered by researchers in the field. The fact that extensive immobilisation decreases bone mass is well known. The determinants of bone structure are a healthy diet with calcium, physical activity and the influence of the reproductive and endocrine systems.

Athletes generally have a bone mass greater than non-athletes. Compared to sedentary individuals, runners are shown to have a higher bone density in their femurs. Tennis players have a greater bone mass in the dominant hand than in the unused hand. Swimmers have lower bone density than athletes involved in land sports such as basketball.

In a yogic practitioner, the general appearance of the skeleton is the same after many years of practice, while in the athlete it appears thicker and bulky. If the athlete deconditions, the wastage is pronounced, and the difference is felt more than when a yogic practitioner stops practising.

Persons who swam regularly had a higher bone density on the vertebral column. In yoga, forward bends, twisting poses and back bends provide a similar effect on the vertebral column. While a person with unhealthy bones, as in Paget's disease, might suffer if dynamic exercises are practised, yoga is safe as the stresses laid are of a different quality.

Post-menopausal women on a training programme, with loads on the wrist and forearm, developed an increase in bone density. It is not surprising that the effects of muscle training have an impact on the bone. In fact, as the bone and muscle are in close contact, it is inevitable that the movement of the muscles affects the bones, like water flowing on rocks affects the surface of the stone.

Yogic preceptors had an intuitive understanding of the human body and had stated ages ago that the skeleton becomes stronger by regular exercise. In asana practice, the muscles actually massage the bones and do not pound the surface. This maintains the health of the bones even without the need for aerobic exercise. Whatever anatomical bony model is provided by nature, yoga maintains the health of this to a ripe old age.

In athletic training, due to the tremendous increases in the stresses laid on the bone, the various anatomical impressions are deeper and more pronounced. No doubt the bones are strong, but yogic training also maintains this strength without the need to pound the bones. For example, the use of standing poses makes the lower limbs so strong that, often, even athletes find it difficult to perform the poses, though their bones are sturdier.

The use of balancing poses places loads on the body different from isometric exercises. The variation in the load is so much that every part of the body is subjected to constant stress, stimulating the bones to remain healthy throughout life. In balancing poses, the stress on all parts of the body is simultaneous, unlike in sporting events where the load distribution depends on the type of sport. Stress fractures occur when the bone under stress cracks without overt strain applied to it. This is a result of habitual stress on the same point, usually in the wrong manner. This is more common in individuals who begin training after middle age and are not given proper guidance about their programme. Fractures have been associated with all kinds of sporting events like tennis, rowing, baseball, throwing events, running and swimming. Habitual walkers suffer from stress fractures of the metatarsal, especially the third.

Stress fractures of the lower extremities are the most common and comprise approximately 95 per cent of the whole. The femoral neck constitutes around 10 per cent of the lower limb fractures. Bone scintigraphy is a very sensitive test to detect early stress fractures and is usually positive 24 hours after the fracture. Any bone in the body can be involved, depending upon the nature of the stress and the type of sport.

The nature of stimulus to the muscles is a dynamic, repetitive, jerky stretch. This ultimately makes the muscles stiff and the athlete is forced to 'warm up' every day. Even though the athlete is in peak form, he or she frequently suffers from muscle, tendon and ligament disorders. The physiological stimulus of a muscle, when subjected to a stretch, is one of reflex contraction, similar to that of an elastic band. This is an inbuilt reflex to prevent a tear. When the stimulus is jerky, the end result is that the muscle contracts and remains shorter than it was at first.

A yoga practitioner never needs to warm up to achieve the most difficult pose, as the body is ever responsive due to the controlled, conscious, integrated type of stretching and contraction stimuli applied. As the nature of stimulus is different, none of the adaptive changes that occur in the body of the athlete occur in the yoga practitioner. A healthy muscle should have a balance between softness and hardness, between rigidity and flexibility. Excessive flexibility is as harmful as rigidity.

Muscles subjected to repetitive movements become hard and nodular over the years. This is in contrast to the body of a yogic practitioner, where the tissues are soft and supple; yet a healthy hardness is maintained. The resting tone of the athlete's muscle is high, while that of the yogic person is at the optimum.

The athlete is never as flexible as the yogi as the training is different. It is essential to have a great deal of flexibility, if the sportsperson is to perform for an extended period of time without occupational hazards. In sports training, isometric and isotonic stresses are given, and the importance of flexibility programmes is recognised to a greater extent today. As a sportsperson needs endurance, speed and stamina of a different kind than normal, the muscles necessarily harden.

A normal individual should ensure that the muscular system can function at a ripe old age as it functioned in childhood. This is ensured by the practice of yoga where the blood supply is maintained, flexibility and rigidity ensured, and load-bearing capacity helped by the balancing poses. The moment the athlete starts practising yoga, he or she realises the difference.

Today, many professional sports-persons all over the world are practising yoga and are realising the benefits in terms of fewer injuries and less fatigue to their systems. In athletic training, muscles exhaust their glycogen store and the build-up of lactic acid is excessive. The type of demand made on the muscles is one of alternating stimulation and fatigue, repetitively, and this, in the long run, produces obvious signs of wear and tear in the system. The necessary changes in the muscle tissue occur where the number of mitochondria alter, and the muscles learn to function for a longer duration even anaerobically. In muscles trained athletically, or with body building gadgets, the arteries and veins are compressed by the very muscles that are developed.

Depending upon the kind of body activity, there are two types of muscle fibres that are used. Activities needing speed recruit fast moving but easily fatiguable muscles, and those needing strength, but not speed, employ slow moving fibres.

The muscles of the sprinter have increased levels of glycogen, adenosine triphosphate (ATP) which is the basic energy molecule of a cell, phosphorylase phosphofructokinase, and increased activity of metabolic reactions that ensure fast and adequate supply of glucose to the working muscle.

Depending upon the nature of the sport, athletes train their bodies. Strength training causes increase in the muscle bulk, and hypertrophy and hyperplasia occur in the muscles. Biopsies from muscles of professional body builders have shown evidence of muscle regeneration and degeneration as an ongoing process. In the body of the yogic practitioner, such changes do not occur, as the nature of the stimulus is different. Most definitely, the adaptive enzymatic changes found in athletic muscles do not occur, as the manner of exercising is different. There is no need for the body to adapt, since blood flow to all parts of the body is maintained, cellular health is ensured, and all the tissues in the body are kept healthy without any change in parameters like blood pressure and oxygen usage.

Fatigue is another important factor in enduring training. There are several mechanisms by which fatigue occurs. Accumulation of lactic acid, hydrogen ions, phosphate, ammonium ions, exhaustion of the cellular energy molecules, are some. In any case, fatigue does occur, and this is nature's built-in reflex to protect the system. The other important factor is the role of the mind in fatigue.

In spite of physiological exhaustion, the power of the mind in influencing the body to achieve is something that modern medicine recognises but cannot explain. Yogic science has always been insisting that the mind is the centre of all power and, if all the reserves of the energy centres in the mind are tapped, fantastic results can be achieved. This explains the yogic powers which are along the lines of the laws of nature. In yogic practice, the kind of fatigue, if it occurs at all, is of a very low grade and the body is flogged in an entirely different manner. In yoga, the accumulation of lactic acid and other metabolites is minimal and does not affect the performance of the joints and muscles.

In athletes, repetitive tears of tendons, ligaments and muscles is a common problem. This is due to the repeated stress of a dynamic nature on the tissues. Fatigue occurs due to constant high intensity and high impact movement, and the ligament or muscle easily tears. Tendons require greater force than muscles to be torn; the fact that this happens is enough proof that strong forces are generated during sporting events. The crux of the matter is that, in sporting events, the body is used like a race horse which has to tire some day, to become a cart horse. Wear and tear occurs if proper servicing is not done.

Evidence of muscle damage has been found in the body of athletes through biopsies which reveal clear elevation of muscle enzymes. When these persons are subjected to high intensity activity, no further increase in the enzyme levels occurs, showing that some sort of adaptation has occurred after extended practice. This is not surprising as the body in sports is subjected to high stress and the system, while producing fantastic results, suffers internally at the same time.

Sportspersons should protect their bodies by practising yoga which soothes the muscles and prevents tears and sprains. It is not good to flog the body. As the movements in sporting events are fast, there is no time for reflection and readjustment to provide for alignment and correct tensions on the joints and muscles. Extension of muscles, bones and joints occurs with tremendous tension in sporting events. But, in yoga, extension occurs without tension due to differences in the manner of training and the logistics of the science.

During yogic practice, a lot of emphasis is placed on alignment and centring, and the movements cannot be classified as isometric or isotonic. The muscle which is contracting at a particular moment of time can be made to stretch, while retaining its contracted state at the same time. This is the peculiarity of yogic movement.

Movement of the muscle tones the joint and improves blood circulation and free flow of nervous energy. In endurance training, the joints are frequently sprained, like the muscles, due to the high intensity of impact and asymmetrical usage. The strain may be mild, moderate, or severe, depending on the type of event; and may vary with individuals, depending on factors like their height and thickness of limbs. The joints are pounded, making the ligaments and joint capsules stiff and non-resilient, and prone to tears and sprains. Even if proper techniques are followed in practising, the nature of the activity is such that injuries result.

Rehabilitation through yoga is necessary as it is the best method to handle joint injuries. Asanas massage the joints and strengthen them along anatomical planes. The joints remain elastic. The shock-absorbing capacity of a joint trained through yoga is far better than with any other system. Flexibility and strength are provided simultaneously. The vast variety in geometric shapes allows different kinds of stresses to be placed on the joints, thus building up maximum health.

In yoga, the joints are moved through seemingly unusual positions; but there is a rational meaning to each position and in no posture are the anatomical tenets broken. All asanas are useful, particularly the standing poses. Padmasana and virasana are valuable for athletes who use their feet often. Hand stand and elbow balance are useful, along with back bends and inversions, for the athlete using the upper limbs.

The female athlete has special problems due to her differing physiology. The training woman has a smaller heart size and heart volume, and higher heart rate, haemoglobin concentration and oxygen content of the blood. Women, in general, have smaller-sized hearts, especially the left ventricle. Blood pressure rises a week prior to the menstrual cycle and starts reducing by day three. Women secrete more catecholamines during exercise, while men do so during non-exercise stresses. A woman also has a smaller lung capacity than a man. There is a sex difference in regulation of skin blood flow which is abolished after menopause.

Due to fat deposits, women may have a greater insulative quality when exercising in the cold. This is offset by a decreased capacity to generate metabolic heat and hence more cooling of the body may occur. Both men and women are similar in their reactions to exercise at high altitudes. The response of circulating lipoproteins to exercise appears to be greater in post-menopausal than in pre-menopausal women; and this suggests that estrogen in the pre-menopausal years is somehow cardio-protective.

Endurance training affects the reproductive system. Menarche occurs later in athletes than in non-athletes. Athletic training could impair the mineralisation of pubertal bone due to the high stress on the muscles, or delay the onset of the menstrual cycle. The amenorrhoea in female athletes is linked to the effects of training. The pituitary hypothalamic axis is affected by training and this in turn affects ovulatory mechanisms.

Improper nutrition is another factor that upsets the reproductive system. The female athlete may suffer three-fold problems—poor nutrition to maintain the ideal body weight, consequent amenorrhea and osteoporosis. A pragmatic view is essential to prevent all these disorders from taking root. In recent years, more women have taken to activities like body building. While the female contour is lost, it is also highly likely that their biological functions will be affected. While one part of the body may benefit by a particular activity, other parts will be adversely affected.

Side Effects of Sports

Injuries occur to sportsmen as the body is subjected to high stresses. The injuries vary according to the kind of sport played and how careful the sportsperson is. Unless early action is taken, the side effects can be disabling. The practice of yoga is of great value to a sportsperson in that it not only helps to prevent the side effects, but also sets them right and maintains the physique. Regarding injuries, the use of plaster casts, crepe bandages, analgesics and rest are useful according to the condition. Yet, this is so only up to a certain point. When the affected part is healed, asana practice is to be instituted as early as possible.

Running

The incidence of injuries varies according to whether the runner is a professional or an amateur. Adequate importance is not given to training in flexibility programmes. Some individuals suffer from anatomical imbalances like flat feet, short legs, excessively lengthy spine, bow legs, knock knees, all of which have to be taken into account when flexibility programmes are introduced. Changes in training schedules, with too much addition all at once, and cross country running are some of the other factors.

In running, foot suffers from repetitive high strain and, in the long run, it suffers from muscular imbalance, losing its arch. The fat pad at the heel wears away and inflammation of the tissues of the sole occur. Spur formation occurs in the heel bone. Stress fractures are very common, with few symptoms, or there can be constant pain unrelieved by training.

Women athletes have to be screened carefully as they are particularly prone to demineralisation of the bones. Constant impact wears the ankle. Recurrent sprains are common and the injury lasts a while. Poor footwear and ill-fitting shoes are other factors that can cause injuries. Inflammation of the achilles tendon is frequent. Athletes cannot stretch the tendon properly in asanas.

The knee is a usual site of affliction accounting for 30 per cent to 40 per cent of injuries. As running is a high impact movement, and one of constant pounding, the wear and tear rate is accelerated. More than tears of the cartilage, the extensor mechanism of the knee is frequently sprained. The quadriceps muscle suffers recurrent sprains. Inflammation occurs in the patellar tendon as it absorbs the constant impact of the pounding force.

Athletes with *genu varum* (bow legs) or *genu valgum* (knock knees) are more affected than others, as the weight transmission is along different lines instead of the perpendicular pathway. The inner surface of the patella and the anterior surface of the femur on which it rests are prone to friction and inflammation. This can lead to premature wear and tear of the structures.

Stiff lower backs and cervical spines are very common in runners. The hip joint is also affected to some extent as the inner groin muscles are frequently sprained. Imbalance in training leads to unequal development of the hip joint muscles and the overdeveloped side suffers pain. The more frequent site of pain is the lower back, even with proper training. This is not surprising, as the lumbar spine is the recipient of compressive stresses that are transmitted by the heavy pounding action.

In order to absorb the impact, the muscles contract at the moment of impact and, with constant use, remain tight all the time. This leads to chronic stiffness and pain, and a sudden movement tears the fascia and the disc. Even these injuries are tolerated by the sportsperson as the mind is conditioned to bear a high degree of pain.

Around nine per cent to 12 per cent of long distance runners suffer from low back pain. These compressive forces can affect the disc and thus affect spinal height. Loss of fluid from the disc has been shown to be the cause of spinal shrinkage. The speed of the run is the main factor that affects the spine.

Though all these problems are commonly found in running, there is an important, often forgotten factor, which is not felt consciously. This is the chemical adaptive change in the muscles of the runner, especially the marathon type. As it is an unnatural state of the body, this sort of change is not good in the long run.

The heart and lungs are 'irritated' by the sport. The stimulus is 'noisy' and does not provide the cellular tranquillity that yoga does. In this sense alone, all exercises are termed irritative. Yoga can also irritate the organs but the nature of the irritation is different. Cardiovascular fitness is built up by running, but this is at the cost of adaptive changes in the heart, muscles and diaphragm.

In women, the reproductive system is affected, resulting in amenorrhoea in some cases. The abdominal organs are disturbed by the constant movement which causes cramping of the circulatory flow.

Yoga is a non-irritative method of stimulation. Running reflects the human potential to achieve. The athlete should not discontinue the sport, but should take precautions to prevent injuries. The flexibility programmes offered to runners today are often done without alignment. Practice of yoga with alignment protects the athlete from all damage. The principal components of yoga improve the shock-absorbing capacity of the system, soften the unhealthy areas and harden the areas where such stimuli are needed.

A strong nervous system is essential for the runner. Intervals of rest followed by training are not correct. Yoga gives rest to the system, allowing better performance. Rest need not mean cessation of activity.

Though the runner's legs are very strong, they are not as stretched as in yoga. Their muscles become more resilient after yogic training and they can run without repeated sprains and tears. A yogic practitioner may not be able to run like an athlete and an athlete finds it difficult to practise asanas. But, as the athlete needs to run, he or she can use yoga and a balance can be brought about between the toughness of the tissues due to running and the resilience of yoga. The cartilages which are constantly pounded by the impact of the run are strengthened and massaged. The hamstring muscles which are tough and hard due to hours of running are softened by the stretches. Likely tears are prevented.

Problems of anatomical disproportion are corrected by asanas. The arches are strengthened and chances of stress fractures are reduced, as the bones are subjected to a different type of stress which protects them. The achilles tendon is made elastic and tears never occur if yoga is practised. The dog pose is particularly valuable as it stretches the achilles tendon. Asanas such as trikonasana, with the heel pushed into the wall, hanumanasana, and seated forward bends with the foot dorsiflexed, are invaluable for this. Cramps in the calf muscles are also relieved by these asanas. Standing in uttanasana with the foot on the semicircular brick, and standing poses done with the heel pushed into the wall are all invaluable for the calf muscles.

The tibia is another area where stress builds up to the extent that many runners suffer from sore muscles on the front of the bone. Practice of virasana removes the pain from the muscles. Runners, walkers and joggers can suffer from the compartment syndrome. There is, in between some muscles in the legs, a strong partition known as fascia. This provides a kind of anatomical division between muscles. As exercising muscles need space to function, and as they bulge if the fascia is not elastic, the bulge of the muscle causes pain and swelling, and limits further movement. Surgery is not needed at all, as yoga has several asanas which can strech the fascia to provide permanent relief.

The shock-absorbing capacity of the knees and ankles can be protected by different positions of virasana cycle. The knee joints are greatly benefited by the practice of virasana, as the opposing surfaces of the femur and the tibia are removed from contact and the cartilages are relieved from the stress of the pounding action.

Padmasana gives great relief from the trauma of the run and one can actually feel the relaxation as it is being practised. Both padmasana and virasana squeeze different parts of the knee joints with a massaging action. This action specifically relieves the impact of pounding stresses. The patella-femoral articulation is prone to developing inflammation, and this is prevented by virasana and padmasana.

Even after inflammation has developed, the asanas relieve pain. If there is a tear in the cartilage, there is no need to rush to surgical management. In the majority of cases, conservative management with yogic exercises is enough to bring the athlete back to normalcy. The injury eventually heals with fibrosis, and any instability or loss of strength can be prevented by the regular practice of asanas.

The quadriceps muscle can be kept healthy by asanas like hanumanasana, virasana and its variations in different positions of standing, kneeling and prone. The hip joint and the groin are closely associated in movement. Any tear of the groin muscle, which is common in athletes, renders effective usage of the hip difficult. All standing poses, asanas like supta padangusthashana with the leg stretched on the side, upavishta konasana and baddha konasana, are invaluable for the athlete.

A common mistake that the majority of sportspersons make is to overstretch the inner groin muscles in baddha konasana, resulting in sprains which do not heal well. Even if they achieve flexibility, it is with a certain quality of rigidity at the same time. Forward bends provide excellent flexibility for the inner groin muscles, which remain resilient and flexible as the movement of bending forward starts from the inner pubic muscles.

A majority of athletes suffer from back pain at some time or another. This is due to lack of forward flexibility. The suppleness in the forward direction is made possible by muscles of a resilient nature. In athletes, the muscles remain hard. Proper practice of basic back bends like urdhva dhanurasana and viparita dandasana results in a very strong bony column, resistant to wear and tear. All the other asanas are also useful. The sportsperson finds it difficult to make the back concave in the standing concave poses.

Due to the constant stoop assumed in training, the dorsal spine develops a hunch. The muscles become hard and inelastic. Proper practice of back bends, especially on the ropes, helps correct the situation. Forward bends done on the wall with the body hanging on the ropes, with the heels on the wall as in either hanging uttanasana or hanging paschimottanasana, help to loosen the muscles in a very short period. Practice of standing poses with the horse prop is important for the athlete to learn the intricacies of alignment and achieve better stability in the body.

The trapezius and the muscles of the shoulder and arm are tightened in the maximum effort achieved during the run. This prevents proper shock absorption and the muscles become hard. Sprains and aches are the most common complaints. Correction of the running technique and practice of inverted asanas like head stand and shoulder stand give the necessary strength and suppleness to the neck and trapezius areas. The heart and lungs are rested periodically by supta virasana.

Paranayama helps to develop stamina. Kumbhakas are useful to develop energy. In the state of retention, the energy drawn in is retained to be properly stored and circulated. If the lungs are exhausted, pranayama in the supine position with pillows refreshes the athlete. Excess heat in the body is removed by sitali pranayama. This is valuable for the marathon runner. The heart and lungs are protected by back bends and forward bends. The abdominal organs are also toned by asanas like supta virasana, purvottanasana, twistings and back bends. Women athletes, who are prone to suffer from amenorrhoea due to high intensities of practice, will benefit from inversions and back bends. The ovaries are stimulated by back bends, and if the uterus is at fault, the forward bends help bring on the flow.

The jumps

Movements in various jumps are always done in a manner that uses one leg excessively.

A high jumper, uses the left or right leg to jump off the ground, and the body is tilted to one side in the process. The repeated use of the same side of the body results in asymmetry, and aches and pains start. The groin muscles are opened only on one side and the hip joints are also subjected to a one-sided strain.

In the case of the long jumper, the launch is with the same leg day after day, and that leg alone is the stronger of the two; similarly with the hip joint and the paraspinal muscles of the back. The hamstrings of one leg are used excessively, while the other leg is passive.

In the triple jump, the person uses one leg to hop and step, and the last part is more strenuous than the long jump, the strain always being on the other leg.

Practice of using both sides of the body should be inculcated in athletes as soon as training is started. Unless ambidexterity is achieved, the body suffers. Bilateral training is a matter of practice and can be achieved. Standing poses help achieve equilibrium in ambidextrous faculties. Right or left handedness in children is only a matter of conditioning and not due to dominant hemispheres. In childhood, any hand can be trained to dominate.

Asanas which open up the groin like upavishta konasana and baddha konasana, samakonasana and supta padangusth-asana, are very useful to prevent imbalances. Hanumanasana optimises muscle usage in the triple and the long jumper. The pole vaulter stresses the muscles of one hand, usually the left, to vault over the bar. The deltoids and the triceps of the left hand are overused. The body is also twisted only to one side to achieve the final jump. The only way to counter these unequal stresses is to train the body on both sides. While this may seem impractical for sport, it is very necessary for health.

Balancing asanas are useful for the vaulter to train both sides of the body for load bearing. One-sided balances like vasishtasana and kasyapasana train the sides of the body and the latissimus dorsi muscles. Asanas which are done dynamically with jumps, with coordination of breathing, are useful to the jumper.

The throws

In throwing sports, arm are the much used body part. In the arm only a few muscles are used all the time and, in the long run, the imbalance between the overused and under-used muscles gives trouble.

In throwing the discus, the palm of one hand is constantly folded, and the other palm is not used. The muscles on the palm are always compressed. The arm that throws is used with a violent fling, and this overstretches the outer triceps and the deltoid junction, and the bottom of the inner armpit area along with the chest. In course of time, the muscles become loose. If stretched over the head, the used arm will move better than the unused arm. The trapezius and the latissimus dorsi are also overstretched, making the used shoulder and the side of the neck appear longer and broader. The real discrepancy is seen when such an athlete performs the asanas.

The ease with which the used arm stretches in the movements is grossly visible. Movements to stretch the palm and improve blood circulation are essential. The athlete will benefit if training is given to both sides of the body. Standing poses correct imbalance on both sides of the body. Asanas like adhomukha svanasana, hand stand, elbow balance, sarvangasana with its variations in arm positions, head stand with its variations in hand positions, different kinds of balancing postures are useful for athlete to redress imbalance of usage.

To a javelin thrower the biceps are more strained in this event, the angle of throw being different. The shoulder joint is violently pulled from the socket along with the scapular muscles. The asanas that help the javelin thrower are the same as for the discus event. In addition, the practice of the reverse namaste removes any soreness from the shoulder joint by internally rotating the joint and the associated muscles of the hand.

In shotput throw, the maximum strain is given to the shoulder joint and associated muscles and ligaments. The heavy fling causes overstretching of the ligaments and muscles. The effects often last for years after cessation of the sport.

In hammer throw the strain on a single hand is less. The shoulder is dragged forcibly. The constant momentum built up before the throw somewhat keeps the arms ready for the event, unlike in the other two events where the arm is kept stationary and then suddenly pushed forward.

The most common problem in the throw events is that of the spine being rotated always to the right. The excessive strain on the facet joints results in an uneven and premature wear and tear and a scoliotic deformity. Lateral bends and twisting asanas are useful to prevent the strain on the spine and maintain healthy evenness of usage. Pranayama, with emphasis on exhalation, is important as the throw will be easier during the exhalation.

Football

Football's effects on the knee are far from simple. Tears in the semilunar cartilage are far more common in this than in any other sport. The knee is rotated outward, with the additional strain of weight bearing. Add to this a sudden jerky movement, and the torsional forces tear the meniscus. The tear can heal by fibrosis. If the tear is large, the knee is prone to sudden locking, the most common complaint.

The player tries to stretch the flexed leg and the movement is halted midway, suddenly and painfully, due to the torn part of the cartilage getting jammed between the femur and the tibia as they glide over each other to complete the stretch of the knee. The cartilage can also become torn through its full length. The typical history is of an acute twisting strain, followed by a sudden feeling of something tearing in the joint and the leg buckling. Effusion of fluid occurs and the patient has to rest in bed for a few days. Once the swelling subsides, activity can be resumed. But the same problem can occur again suddenly, without warning, with the knee buckling.

The usual routine of physiotherapy exercises is not of much value as the movements are dynamic and irritative to the inflamed tissues. The range of movement in yoga is far more, and the nature of load bearing is different. Relief of pain occurs within a few days of therapy. The synovial thickening may take longer to thin down. The resisted exercises which are used in physiotherapy are not very helpful in the long run as inflammation can increase.

Yoga also uses resisted exercises, but the nature of loading is different. Yoga does not provide mechanical, repetitive, movements. It is improper to classify yoga as isometric, as both isometric and isotonic strains are given to a muscle at a single point in time. All standing poses are important. Each tones up a different portion of the knee joint and the stress and strain offered by each pose is different. Standing poses strengthen, realign and massage the cartilages and improve weight bearing. The use of the foot rest with the foot dorsiflexed and the knee locked, and the ascension of the quadriceps strengthen the knee.

Alignment is very important in performing these poses. This concept is absent in physiotherapy exercises. Inversions teach proper alignment of the knees which is much more difficult to achieve in the standing poses. The muscles become strong as the anti-gravity action is used. Variations are also helpful. Padmasana and virasana, with their massaging actions, are highly beneficial to tone up the cartilages. The supporting muscles of the knee joint are also made flexible and massaged. This relieves pain. Back bends educate the knee in the most difficult way. As it is more difficult to direct and control the muscles of the knee in these poses, great skill is needed. Supta virasana preceded by viparita karani relieves the strain of constant running.

Hockey

A hockey player has to bend to one side all the time during tackling. The spine is always inclined to the side; one arm extended, the other contracted. The dominant shoulder is overstretched; the inner biceps and forearm muscles are taxed. The legs are also used asymmetrically with more stress on the rear knee. The spine is laterally turned to the right and rotated to the left. Flexion of the spine is a constant accompaniment with the need to run about continuously. In the long run, problems of low back ache, wear and tear of the knees and, the cervical muscles occur.

Dog pose is ideal to correct the imbalances in the spinal muscles. The knees also become stronger in the process. Standing poses done to correct the tilt and rotation are necessary. Virasana and padmasana are useful to rest the overused knees. Inversions help overcome exhaustion and, when combined with supta virasana, relieve fatigue of the leg muscles at the end of the day. Viparita karani can also be combined with supta virasana. Virasana with a pillow between the knees also gives relief to tired legs. Back bends like urdhva dhanurasana and viparita dandasana are helpful to induce symmetry of posture and movement in the hands and shoulders.

Cricket

As the world's most popular game, cricket is becoming very rough today. Players have to use headgear and other protective devices to shield themselves from injury. Awareness of the need for prematch conditioning is greater than before.

Right-handed batsmens have to constantly bend the body forward and incline the spine and the eyes to the left. The left hip always projects along with the left shoulder. The right shoulder is always lower than the left and the clavicular area is hollowed out on the left. Asanas which work on the knees, turn the spine to the right, push the hip to the right, open the right shoulder and flatten the clavicular area are to be practised. Forward bends cool the body which is exposed to the sun for long hours. Long hours of standing will be relieved by performing viparita karani on the wall, followed by supta virasana with pillows under the thighs. Back bends give the batsman the energy needed to play for many hours without tiring. Use of props at the end of a long day refreshes the player for the next day.

Bowlers also suffer from hand, spinal, knee and ankle problems and exhaustion from constant running. The entire spine is always turned to one side, with or without force. The trapezius of the non-dominant shoulder is constantly contracted and this forms a nodule in the long run. The cervical muscles are turned to the same side all day, and rotational asymmetry occurs.

The knee and ankle on the non-used side can take excess weight at the time of completing the movement. Before this phase the bowler has to lean back on the other knee and the inner ligament can suffer strain. This is repeated for years. Excessive wear and tear of the spine occurs and can cause degenerative changes. All standing poses are helpful for the spine, knee and ankle.

Trapezius traction relieves the pain in the shoulder and the nodule can be shrunk. Rotational movements such as standing marichyasana and bharadwajasana give relief to the neck. Extension of the neck on the rope, holding the bar behind the back, and back bends with rope give relief to the neck and the shoulders.

Hand stand and elbow stand are useful to provide extension for the hands. Inversions, forward and back bends are all needed. Back bends give the necessary endurance to the pace bowler. As the bowler has to move constantly, resting poses like viparita karani, forward bends on the pillows, virasana and its cycle are all very helpful. Virasana is particularly useful for the knees and ankles.

Wicket keepers have to squat and rise several hundred times daily. This can lead to fatigue of the spinal muscles and groin muscles, and produce low back and cervical aches due to constant flexion and extension of the neck with overusage. The hips and the knee joints also face the same strain. The groin muscles are semi-open, retarding healthy blood flow in those areas. The organs of perception are also overused as the keeper has to study the movement of the ball and be very alert. The wicket keeper has to practise all asanas to prevent the back from premature degeneration. Back bends give enormous relief to the entire anterior and posterior spine.

Inversions give respite from the constant congestion in the legs due to squatting, which prevents healthy venous return and fresh arterial flow. They also help the neck by flexing it, particularly half halasana and shoulder stand. Hamstring stretches as in the standing poses and supta padangusthasana, samakonasana and hanumanasana are relieving to the muscles which are constantly flexed. Baddha and upavishta konasana assuage the strain on the groin along with supta baddha konasana. Forward bends and half halasana soothe the senses. Practice of shanmukhi mudra is useful to lighten strain on the mind and the eyes.

Fielders are not suffering so much from postural problems. Close quarter fielders flex their spine, hips and knees constantly. Practice of asanas is as for the wicket keeper. Exposure to the sun and loss of fluid and salts deplete energy. Passive inversions and supta virasana are helping to relieve from fatigue.

All pranayamic techniques are useful for cricket players. In short, the practice of yoga makes a perfect cricketer.

Wrestling

Wrestling has been forced to become harsh today. There are many styles and a common factor is that the body has to be fattened and kept heavy. Body contact being inevitable, injuries result. The mildest variation is surno wrestling, where the aim is to push the person out of the ring. Surno wrestlers, being grossly overweight, suffer from diabetes, hypertension and premature degenerative disorders of the spine, hip, knee and ankle joints. The sensitivity of the body suffers due to overeating, which assumes enormous proportions. Once the person retires the inactivity, combined with the overweight, destroys the body very easily.

Wrestlers frequently use various diet methods, such as fasting, vomiting, laxatives, diuretics, sauna, rubber sweat-suits, or heated wrestling rooms. Some of these methods induce weight loss by dehydration. The wrestler has been known to gorge on food and fluid after the event, only to repeat the process of weight control for the next selection event. All this is extremely harmful to the body metabolism. Natural methods of weight maintenance are healthier.

All body parts of the wrestler are stiff. Wrestlers often cannot squat on the ground or raise their arms freely overhead. The weight of the body combined with bulk of fat prevents healthy movements. The right perspective towards this event is to avoid fattening the body at all and use safe techniques while fighting. All asanas are useful. Standing poses protect the knees and hip joints.

Weightlifting

The muscles of the weightlifter increase in size and cross sectional area. This is an adaptive situation. Yet it is unhealthy, as the other organs are affected in the process and the stress induced is asymmetrical on the body. Weightlifting is a strong stimulus for bone formation and mineralisation. Endurance training does not produce such increases. The weightlifter has to have a high calorie diet to qualify for certain categories. Manipulating dietary factors might be harmful to the body. The heavier the weight lifted, the brighter the chances of topping the competition.

Although the weightlifter can bear enormous loads, the excess weight gained is a constant strain on the heart, lungs and abdominal organs. The arms are out of proportion to the rest of the body and strained excessively, especially when the person strives to break records. The increase in the intra-abdominal pressure is transmitted to the back and, if a belt is not worn, a ruptured ligament or disc often results. Chronic low back pain due to injury during training, and overusage due to excessive loading, are usual.

The weightlifter has to wear knee and ankle caps to protect the joints. The thigh muscles are overdeveloped in lifting heavy loads. The joints of the lower limbs always turn outward at the moment of lifting. This can affect the medial ligaments of the ankles, knees and hips.

The left ventricular mass is greater in weightlifters, related to the maximum aerobic capacity. Due to the compression of the intra-thoracic organs during the lift, the left ventricle can undergo hypertrophy in response to persistent loading. The blood pressure can rise to enormous levels at the time of the lift. The lungs are also compressed, hindering free mechanisms of inspiration and expiration in the long run. The shoulders and the accessory muscles of the neck tighten, breathing is laboured and the diaphragm tight, the eyes congested.

The entire cardiorespiratory system is always under tremendous tension. Due to the rise in intra-abdominal pressure, the organs are compressed and the cells are kept in a 'shrunken state' with reduction in blood circulation. The gall bladder, liver and pancreas are pressurised. The abdominal aorta is pressed. Colonic pressure can rise to several times more than normal. The kidneys and pelvic organs are stressed.

A weightlifter may be strong but circulatory and nervous energies cannot flow freely in such a person. Movements should be graceful and light, not heavy and sluggish. Practice of yoga is highly beneficial. The even usage of the body during asanas prevents regional over-stimulation of the bone. The neck and arms are benefited by inversions, hand stand, dog pose done both ways, and elbow stand. The elbows and wrists are kept well aligned and supple by urdhva hastasana, reverse namaste, dog pose, hand and elbow stand. The mid and lower back and the ligaments and muscles of the lower limbs are kept soft and supple by standing poses. The use of the horse prop is essential to help the heavy weightlifter perform the standing poses. As the muscles may be oversized and stiff, it may be physically impossible in some persons to achieve flexibility without the prop. The twisting poses are very valuable for softening the hardened muscles of the weightlifter. Back bends done passively relieve strain on the back by giving rest to the posterior muscles of the spine. Forward bends improve blood supply to the posterior spinal muscles which are always constricted during weightlifting. The strain on the heart, circulation, blood pressure and the lungs is prevented by regular practice of standing and seated forward bends, in a modified way to suit the lifter. Forward bends done passively with the bandage relieve strain on the senses and the sympathetic nerves. Back bends promote excellent expansion of the intra-thoracic organs. The diaphragm, which is hard in weightlifters, is softened by back bends and twisting poses.

The pelvic organs, which are pressurised in the squatting position, get relief from baddha and upavishta konasana. It is difficult to rationally integrate yoga and weightlifting for persons interested in both the arts, for the mechanisms are different; but the practice of yoga is needed to prevent the side effects of the latter.

Gymnastics

Gymnastics is one of the most graceful sporting events but it has another side. We may not be aware of the stress on the body in the training period and the effect, during the pre-pubertal years, on the healthy growth of the body and on menarche in females.

The gymnast suffers later in life when it is difficult to reverse many of the side effects. Weight has to be kept constant and this can affect the nutritional status and the reproductive system. Female gymnasts have broad shoulders like a male and the pronounced female curve of the hips is lacking. This is due to training the body at too young an age. The shoulders are broader and most teenage female gymnasts show poor breast development. Though studies have shown that the small stature of the gymnasts is more often due to selection than the effects of training, premature high intensity training on the delicate cartilages and joint junctions of the child is not advisable. The strong traction forces working on the unossified bones can hinder proper development. When a bone's capacity to repair itself is overcome by such strong forces, stress fractures result.

Male gymnasts are also narrower in the lower half of the body. The arms tend to be overdeveloped. The most detrimental aspect of the training is that of imposing excessive flexibility and loads on tender bodies. Yet another factor is that of constant back bend practice. Most of the time the performance of gymnasts is punctuated with extension movements. The stretching movements of the spine and the legs are often done without proper alignment. This leads to ligaments and muscles that are looser than normal. Sprains of the lower lumbar muscles are common. The spine is constantly bent backwards.

Knee disorders due to outward turn of the foot during movements are common. Jerky movements are used for the upper arms and lower limbs. Hence, recurrent injuries to the wrists, knees and ankles force the gymnast to wear ankle and knee braces to maintain stability. There is often no time for the gymnast to adjust the joints and muscles and optimise the load to different parts of the body. Moreover, during performances, the mind is under great tension. The same person performs better under non-competitive practice conditions. This problem is common for all performance artists, but in the case of the gymnast the consequence could be serious physical injury.

Yoga helps gymnasts to learn the principles of alignment in stretching and contracting the muscles, joints and ligaments of the body. It helps them to understand how to balance movements of extension and flexion for all parts of the body. Refinement of the intelligence with regard to the body and mind through yoga is useful. Pranayama is useful to relieve stress on the mind and senses.

By yoga the gymnast can ensure that every cell is in alignment and then balanced. Poise is constantly refined every day, in the same pose, so that stagnation never occurs. Hand stand and elbow stand help in the proper alignment of the arms. The spine, hip and the knee joints suffer premature wearing, which can be prevented by standing poses. The gymnast learns the right method of alignment by these poses.

Inversions are useful to give rest from the stress of performances, and forward bends quieten the senses and also allow better stabilisation of the body which is constantly bent backwards. Back bends give endurance both to the body and the mind, and, along with setubandha sarvangasana on the props, rest to the mind during emotional depression. Back bends done in the way of gymnastics constitute hyper-extension of the spine. The gluteal muscles are not used. The dorsal spine is not used properly. Yoga teaches the correct geometry of these poses to the gymnast.

Alignment of baddha and upavishta konasana, and samakonasana along with hanumanasana have to be understood carefully by the gymnast. The manner of the gymnastic split is imprecise as the sciatic nerve is under pressure due to the wrong position of the piriformis muscles of both the hip joints. Yogic techniques teach the right method of these asanas which prevents injuries.

Cycling

To the cyclist, yoga is very helpful. Hand stand and elbow stand improve blood circulation and remove unnatural strain in the hands. Counter movements are also provided for. The shoulders are stretched by back bends. Standing poses help the lower limbs and spine to remain resilient and supple. The hamstrings derive better blood flow as they are stretched well. Inversions and forward bends 'cool' the 'heated' brain. Back bends open out the contracted chest and stimulate healthy and effortless blood flow in all the organs in the thorax, the abdomen and the pelvis. This stimulates the nervous system.

Baddha and upavishta konasana stimulate blood flow in the pelvic and genital areas and relieve congestion. The genital organs feel revitalised, the practitioner experiencing a sense of warmth and lightness in those areas. Viparita karani and supta virasana with pillows between the calf and thigh muscles are very helpful as the latter massages the tired muscles without any disturbance, giving rest and relief to the aching muscles of the legs. This is particularly valuable in relieving lower limb fatigue. Pranayama is helpful to prevent, onset of fatigue.

Swimming

Swimming precludes the harmful effects of impact as in land sports. A person with a low back disorder can swim easily, as the buoyancy prevents load on the back. Even if the swimmer suffers most of the common orthopaedic disorders of a mechanical nature, swimming never poses difficulties. Yet, there are other problems. The first concern is body weight maintenance. This can, in turn, lead to nutritional deficits.

In women, certain areas tend to be hyperatrophied and overexercised. The excessive usage of the pectoral muscles causes loss of fatty tissue in the breast and most female swimmers show poor breast development. The distribution of the female body fat is also affected and the general contour of the body leans towards that of a male. The leg and calf muscles hypertrophy; the shoulder and posterior thoracic cage muscles enlarge.

The cardiovascular efficiency is as good as in any athlete on land. One of the greatest benefits is the healthy development of respiratory power as the head dips in and out of water. The glandular system can get exhausted with overtraining. The professional swimmer's lipid profile does not appear to undergo any special changes because of swimming.

Even though swimming is considered a non-weight bearing exercise, the density of the radius and vertebral area was higher in men who swam regularly than in those who did not. The increase in bone density is due to the high intensity muscular activity. Professional divers risk injuries to the eyes and neck. The intensity of the impact during diving can affect the retina. The eyes and ears are irritated due to the constant influx of water. The hands and legs are used in a different manner than on land. The intense heat of the muscular activity opens the pores of the skin but, as the water is cool, an inhibiting effect occurs on the sweat gland function.

Yogas like hand stand, dog pose, elbow balance, back bends, teach the proper stretch of the arms and nullify strain. Inversions protect the eyes, sinuses, ears and legs from fatigue. Supta virasana relieves cardiorespiratory fatigue. Forward bends expose the body to the external atmosphere and allow time for healthy perspiration. Back bends make the body sweat to dissipate the internal heat. They also provide stamina. For exhaustion of the legs, viparita karani and supta virasana are valuable. The groins, which are constantly constricted, are benefited by baddha and upavishta konasana. Pranayama helps maintain a healthy coordination between exhalation and inhalation, which is very necessary as the upper respiratory organs dip in and out of water. It prevents stress on the respiratory organs.

Skiing

Since 2500 BC, much sophistication has developed in the availability of gadgets for skiing. The physiological changes in cross-country skiing are similar to endurance training. Here, large groups of muscles are put to work. The amount of oxygen consumed is high. The cardiorespiratory fitness is similar to that of endurance athletes. The heart shows an increase in the thickness of the left ventricular wall. The muscles of the legs, however, are shown to have a lower oxidative capacity than that of long distance runners.

Major areas of stress build-up are hands and shoulders, spine, groin, knees and ankles. The hands are always used in a flexed manner and never stretched out. The shoulders are constantly used in a one-sided manner. The spine is bent forward and, combined with the pressure on the groin, this reduces circulation in the inner organs. All the spinal muscles suffer fatigue. The knees and ankles suffer ligament strains and tears due to the constantly bent position. The situation is worse if a slip occurs. Though high impact is absent, wear and tear of the cartilages occur due to over-usage.

The skier can practise all standing poses to prevent degeneration of the spine and the lower limbs. Inversions combined with supta virasana give relief to aching legs. Baddha and upavishta konasana provide for healthy pelvic blood flow. Hamstring stretches relieve the constantly compressed muscles. The spine is helped by all asanas. Back bends are essential to relieve the stress of the constant stoop and provide cardiorespiratory toning to help prevent easy exhaustion at altitudes. Back bends on the ropes are ideal for the beginner to provide quick relief. Supine pranayama relieves fatigue and to improve endurance all varieties can be practised.

Rowing

In rowing, the parts of the body that suffer are the spine, groin and hands. The constant flexion movement has produced fatigue fractures of the vertebral bodies. Over the years, the spine can suffer premature degeneration due to repeated flexion stresses. The knee may be kept semi-straight or straight and, if the latter, the lumbar region suffers strain. The dorsal spine is excessively bowed. The chest often suffers a caving. The points of the buttock bones become sensitive to pain due to constant pressure. The muscles of the arms face the stress of asymmetrical usage. The action is always of a closed nature and this restricts healthy blood flow in the arms. The heart and lungs, being subjected to the effect of a forward bend, do not enjoy fresh blood flow. The lungs cannot draw in fresh oxygen.

The posture is a load on the circulatory and respiratory systems. The intestine, gall bladder and pancreas are pressurised, restricting the flow of fresh healthy blood in the abdominal aorta. The pelvic organs are compressed and, in the female, undesirable pressure on the ovaries, the uterus and its supporting ligaments is produced. Hand stand, elbow balance and back bends teach proper extension of the arms maintain suppleness and blood flow. They prevent malalignment and overusage of the same group of muscles. Standing poses give relief to the spinal muscles and lower limbs of the oarsman.

Baddha and upavishta konasana open the constricted groin area, improving blood circulation. Inversions cool the brain which is constantly in the flexed position. They also relieve the circulatory stagnation by allowing fresh blood to enter all the inner organs. Setu bandha sarvangasana refreshes the heart, lungs and spinal muscles due to its concave geometry and improves the circulation in the thoracic organs. This gives greater energy to the rower as there is rest to the lungs which can draw in greater quantities of oxygen.

Practice of back bends provides relief to the spinal muscles, the thoracic and intra-abdominal organs. Back bends are very important to relieve the strain of the flexed position both for the skeletal system and the inner organs. Passive back bends on the props are useful to relieve cardiorespiratory fatigue. Pranayama enhances endurance and reduces strain on the sense organs.

Archery

In the sports of archery, one eye and shoulder are strained excessively and one side of the brain is used more than the other. The pull of the arm backwards results in a contraction of the biceps, and stretch of the triceps, and contraction of the scapular muscles. In the arm that pulls the string of the bow, the trapezius muscle that connects the root of the neck to the shoulder joint is made to contract repeatedly.

Over the years, the sportsperson develops a nodule in the trapezius. On the other side, the scapular muscles are stretched along with the latissimus dorsi and the rest of the hand. There is no difference in the occurrence of problems even with modern archery gadgets, where, to a certain extent, some mechanisation has taken place. The neck muscles are also used in a lopsided manner, like the eyes, as they turn to one side constantly.

Hand stand, elbow stand, dog pose done both ways with fingers on the wall and in the opposite direction, balancing poses and unilateral balancing poses like vasishtasana, are useful to achieve balance of both sides of the body including the hands. Forward bends relieve eye strain while back bends provide confidence. The archer must use the unused part of the body more in asana practice so that it compensates for the inactivity during archery. Pranayama of the contemplative type—nadi shodana—is highly useful for the archer who is unable to concentrate. In this, the mind has to quieten, and the sensitivity of the fingertips is honed to trace the passage of the breath.

Shooting

In shooting, the hand positions are similar to archery, except that the left arm is held bent instead of extended. The weight of the gun is different and the recoil varies with the calibre. The butt of the gun digs into the shoulder and, over the years, creates a pressure pain on the inner deltoid muscle. The position also uses the outer deltoids more than the inner. The inner is always stretched. The trapezius on the side of the butt is chronically contracted. The hand that holds the gun from the bottom suffers a contraction of the deltoid, and the triceps and biceps. The usage of the eye is similar in principle to archery.

The asanas that help the archer also help the shooter. For both, the use of the ropes on the shoulder, in the form of a harness, relieves the strain on the trapezius and prevents nodule formation. Dog poses, hand stand, head and shoulder stand with the belt, all relieve elbow and shoulder problems. In both archery and shooting the eyes are strained to the maximum. To relieve eye strain, practice of forward bends, with the bandage on the eyes, and of shanmukhi mudra, is beneficial.

Tennis

In tennis, the serving arm is used excessively by tennis players, producing the speed of the serve. The other arm is grossly underused. The wrist also suffers the same fate. In the well-used wrist, the bones and muscles are firmer and larger. The forearm is thicker on the dominant hand. The rotators of the back are used more towards one side and the vertebrae are twisted always to the same side. The excess stress creates spur formation on the verterbrae.

If the player has a habit of top spinning the ball, the inner elbow and wrist are overused. If the backhand stroke is single handed, the outer forearm and upper arm muscles are preferentially used. If double handed, the inner forearm and upper arm muscles of the helping arm are overused. But, it is the dominant arm that is always overused. The inner elbow is prone to inflammation if the player does not maintain adequate tension of the forearm muscles at the moment of impact, the so-called 'tennis elbow'. The spine and neck are always overly twisted to the opposite side.

If the style of the player is one of over-extension of the spine in reaching for the ball during the serve, the resulting momentum and twist is extreme. The rear knee always takes more weight at the beginning of the serve. The foot on the other side suffers excess weight transmission at the end of the serve. The shoulders are protected by movements in head and shoulder stands. The reverse namaste is valuable to prevent excess wear and tear in the head of the shoulder joint. A good policy is to instil the habit of using both sides of the body even as initial training begins for the novice.

Asanas like hand stand, dog pose including the upward dog, balancing poses, inversions and unilateral balancing poses help relieve any pathology in the shoulder and the elbow. All standing poses help the player to be more limber on court, prevent malalignment and pain problems in different parts of the body. Back bends give the endurance needed as it is common to see players gasping at the end of the serve after many games. Forward bends provide rest for the system, both between and after matches. These can be done with the props if fatigue exists. Viparita karani, followed by supta virasana, is valuable to give the entire neuro-endocrine system rest and recuperation after a match. The ham-strings and the Achilles tendon are kept elastic by asanas like hasta and supta padangusthasana. The knees are protected by virasana and padmasana.

Squash

Squash is a high impact sport. The movement, when the ball is reached for has to be abruptly terminated to move in another direction immediately. As the ball is bounced back from very close quarters, there is very little resting period for the forces of acceleration and deceleration. This results in the knee and the hip and the back absorbing the impact. In the long run, many suffer chronic shoulder pain and knee pain, especially in the region of the medial ligament.

The forces that work on the hand and the shoulder are far greater than in tennis, and the violent swing can injure the ligaments of the shoulder. Tears of the ligament are not uncommon. The high impact on the foot results in strained arches, pain in the soles and flat feet.

Squash is fast and forceful and the nerves get exhausted soon. The entire spine is used asymmetrically and with high impact. The shearing forces on the muscles are very forceful. Sprains of the spinal muscles are common. The shoulder ligaments are prone to becoming overstretched. Reverse namaste, salamba sarvangasana, half halasana and baddha padmasana are useful to retain the tightness of the ligaments. The knee and foot are helped by asanas like virasana which relieve the strain of the impact by their massaging action. It is important to practise resting poses like setu banda sarvangasana and passive forward bends to recover from fatigue.

To protect the spine, standing poses are invaluable. The higher incidence of low back pain is due to the high striking force of the heel at the moment of strike. The usual routine of asanas for low back pain relieves the condition. This includes bharadwajasana near the wall, standing marichyasana, lateral bends like trikonasana, parsvakonasana, dog poses, pawana muktasana and savasana with weights on the lumbar spine to massage the muscles. In spite of adequate precaution, many suffer chronic low back pain and knee disorders. The nature of the game is such.

Yoga does protect the body, but the intensity of the knee strike should be reduced if the knee and back are to remain healthy in the long run. All types of pranayama are useful. Bandhas and kumbhakas are necessary to improve endurance.

Golf

In golf, the wrist is most commonly sprained. The dominant shoulder with the associated muscles are over-contracted. The other hand suffers less. The spine is another area of neglect. As the stroke is completed, the entire spine is turned to the extreme left and, over the years, the rotators of the spine suffer the effects of asymmetric usage. Premature degenerative changes occur, resulting in spondylitis. The knees suffer asymmetrical usage and the rear knee is twisted constantly as the stroke is completed. There is pain in the region of the medial ligament of the knee.

Asanas involving the wrist, like the dog pose, chaturanga dandasana, sarvangasana, halasana and balancing poses, are all useful. The spine and eye muscles can be balanced by all standing poses and twisting asanas near the wall. All other spinal movements can also be practised for complete suppleness. As the golfer has to walk for long hours, virasana with a pillow between the thigh and calf relieves fatigue and pain in the lower limbs. This may be preceded by viparita karani against the wall. Exposure to the sun for long hours produces heat in the body. Forward bends done passively are valuable to cool the system.

Polo

In polo the bend of the spine to the same side occur repeatedly. The load on the spine in this game is considerable as the player has to bend from a height. The left side of the spine is overstretched. The neck muscles are also used lopsidedly. The intercostal muscles on the dominant side are also constantly compressed. The inner groin and the adductors on the dominant side of the thigh are overused. The left groin and adductors are compressed.

Practice of hand stand and elbow balance is needed. The remedy for the spine is to practise lateral bending poses like trikonasana and parsvakonasana, and standing rotational movements like parivrtta trikonasana and parsvakonasana. Parivrtta janu sirsasana is very valuable. Baddha konasana and upavishta konasana are essential to ensure even usage of groin muscles. Back bends are a must, as the spine is always bent forward. These poses also squeeze the kidneys and prevent excess mobility of the organs due to constant riding. To make up for uneven arm usage, practice bouts with the left arm are essential.

Billiards

In billiards the position of the leg, arm, spine and neck is so awkward that postural problems can set in very easily. One leg is sometimes placed back and the other forward, and this automatically tilts the pelvis. One arm and shoulder are stretched forward and the other drawn back, and the elbow constantly bent. The deltoid muscle of the striking hand is contracted in the outer aspect. The arm pit and the wrist of the stretched arm are overused and so is the latissimus muscle of the extended arm.

The trapezius of the extended arm is constantly contracted. The neck and the eyes are forced to look in an awkward manner in relation to the rest of the body. The spine is rotated to the right and tilted to the left or constantly bent forward. One side of the abdomen is contracted and the other side stretched. The legs suffer exhaustion due to long hours of standing.

Standing postures with emphasis on lateral bends to the right side, rotational movements oriented to the left, are all helpful to overcome the constant one-sided usage of the body, along with parivrtta janu sirsasana. Asymmetrical knee and ankle usage is also beneficial. Inversions relieve the long hours of standing and correct the tilt of the neck Posterior hand stretches on the window and the wall ropes, along with hand stand and elbow balance, are essential to relieve the stress of asymmetrical usage.

The practitioner should work the muscles of the deltoid and triceps area of the left hand more consciously than the right side. Both sides of the chest should be attended to in all poses, particularly back bends. If the player is attentive to all this, he or she is less likely to suffer the effects of chronic asymmetrical usage. The stooped posture is similar to practising a half uttanasana always, without countering it. Hence, the person will experience the effects of a semi-forward bend. The organs are always pressed. Back bends are essential to stimulate the lungs and heart, as the body is always bent forward, compressing them. Practice of viparita dandasana on the rack before the match will refresh the mind and the eyes and prevent exhaustion.

Overtraining syndrome

Overtraining syndrome is a physiological condition of excessive and prolonged fatigue in the sportsperson due to exceeding the limits of the training programme, like training at high intensities and without periods of rest. The symptoms include fatigue, loss of weight, elevated blood pressure, rapid pulse rate, digestive dysfunction, insomnia and some emotional disturbances. Studies have demonstrated both elevated and depressed levels of catecholamines in the system.

Sports anaemia is another important factor. Endurance athletes appear to have low iron content in their bodies. This situation can occur with any kind of sporting event. There can be no generalisation as to the limits of endurance permissible for each sport, as each individual is different and guidelines have to be personalised. Modern medicine tries to give a general guideline for all human beings.

Yoga believes in attending to every individual and advising each according to his or her needs. The human body may be the same, but the mind is different and conditioning varies. In addition, there is the problem of the psyche with its innumerable layers of consciousness, all of which play an important role in determining the behaviour of an individual.

The sportsmen are anxious to maintain the status won over years of hard struggle which makes the mind get attached to these achievements. This attachment will lead to agony if the person is not able to maintain this position. In a long career, this continued stress on the mind can cause a nervous breakdown. This is becoming all too common today. In order to avoid this, intense training is needed—for the sportsperson to have an attitude of total detachment from the fruits of labour. Here, yoga can show the way towards mental detachment and consequent freedom. The sports professional should ensure some means of relaxation in daily life. In the pressure of achievement, the individual could lose all spontaneous interest in the game and be involved in it mechanically, as a performing machine. Training centres all over the world must provide an atmosphere of quietitude and opportunities for recuperation.

An athlete should include all nutrient food items in his diet. A balanced diet including all parameters will prevent any undernourishment in the athlete. Ragi is very good as its high calcium and energy content is valuable to the athlete. Food should be easily digestible; food high in carbohydrates is desirable. This is digested the fastest, followed by protein and fat. Adequate energy is the most important requirement of the sportsperson.

Any unused energy is stored as fat in the body. Carbohydrates are the preferential fuel for high intensity work, as they enrich glycogen stores. The recommended daily intake of carbohydrates is around 500 to 600 gm. Ingestion of carbohydrates before and during events has been shown to improve performance. After an event, ingestion of fluids rich in carbohydrates replaces muscle glycogen. The fat content is kept as low as possible to prevent atherosclerosis. Liquid foods are used up faster than solid foods.

Life Expectancy of Athletes

Athletes are basically healthy persons. They have an increased life expectancy because of the high levels of fitness. The factors that enhance lifespan are many and habitual physical activity is only one of them. The others are a healthy diet and minimal stress in one's life in terms of having the right attitude to challenging situations.

It is very common to find yogis in the region of the Himalayas living to over a hundred years and possessing an excellent quality of life. The reason has been attributed to their practice of yogic techniques and serene living. Their stress-free life is not because they are remote from human habitations, but because of their calm approach to life.

The yogis of India never practised endurance exercises, yet their lifespan has been very long. Achieving health is not just due to a single causative factor; it is always a combination of the right diet, adequate exercise and an equanimous attitude to life. Each parameter has its own role to play in human physiology, and health, as mentioned before, is a summation of all three. The human body has a tremendous capacity to adapt to any physiological situation. The yogis in the Himalayan ranges remain at high altitudes for years together, barebodied, without any deleterious effects. The fact that the yogis can control the autonomic functions of their bodies has been observed time and again.

Today's athlete must refrain from consuming any drug that might affect the body, this is ethical discipline towards oneself. The overtraining syndrome must never occur. The practice of athletics must be one of purity in all facets and, when this is strictly followed, satya exists. In the niyamas, saucha is strictly required if the body is to excel in sports. The athlete must strive to maintain the inner purity of the body by practice of yoga, so that the system will serve for a longer period with a healthier quality. Dejection should not be allowed to possess the mind. Tapas are practised, to achieve, one strives with single-minded concentration. In addition to this, if the mind has an inner quietitude, tapas blazes with greater intensity.

Swadhyaya helps an athlete to discover the inherent faults of his body and mind. Unless the reactions of the body and mind are reflected upon and adjustments made, refinement in technique will not result. This faculty of study is a never-ending process to prevent stagnation in practice. In athletics, due to the fast pace of events, there is little time to feel the movement of the individual parts of the body. In yoga, the mind is trained to reflect from moment to moment, but not to be caught in the movement of the moment. The trained mind is in a state of quietness which makes it razor sharp to root out imbalances. This refines the practice.

Pranayama leading to withdrawal of the senses—pratyahara which relieves the mental and physical strain of the athlete. Pratyahara prevents excessive build-up of stress in the body of the sportsperson and removes the hitherto accumulated stress. Stress is ever there, it is needed for proper stimulation of the body and mind.

Dharana, dhyana and samadhi—the last three stages of yoga—help the athlete to bring the body and mind to a state of total poise and stability in all the sheaths. Dharana is always used by all. Yoga teaches the sportsperson to strengthen this faculty when the asanas and pranayama are practised. In yogic practice, the self and the cells are connected. This leads to introspective action. When concentration is refined and is continuous, it becomes meditation. The state of meditation helps the athlete to remain unaffected by results but to act for the moment. This merges into samadhi, through which athletes perform without being affected in any manner, physically or mentally.

AGING AND YOGA

Aging cell has a poorer capacity to remove the normal amount of free radicals formed in the body. Retention of free radicals is toxic to the body. The dwindling capacity is multifactorial—stress, poor nutrition, unhealthy living and lack of exercise. Antioxidants try to counter the existence of free radicals and slow the aging process. The three most important antioxidants are superoxide dismutase, catalase and glutathione peroxidase. Aging of the cells is associated with a decline in protein synthesis and cellular proliferation, thus affecting the turnover of antioxidants.

With aging, coronary arteries become blocked with plaques, reducing coronary flow. This can lead to a heart attack resulting in death of the tissue. The size of the capillaries in the skeletal muscles diminish, and muscle blood flow is reduced. The elasticity of the blood vessels weakens, adding to flow reduction. This increased tension in the peripheral vessels causes an increase in blood pressure and reflex strain on the heart. The heart has to pump harder to maintain a healthy circulation.

As the cells do not derive a healthy supply of blood, retention of cellular toxins damages the tissues. Calcification of major and minor blood vessels occurs, much depending on the diet, age and sex, physical activity, level of atmospheric pollution and genetic predisposition to the condition. Atherosclerosis, which means hardening of the arteries with resultant reduction in blood flow to the affected area, is a major killer in the world today. The arch of the aorta becomes calcified. All blood vessels in the body undergo degeneration, particularly in the heart and brain. Intramuscular reduction in blood flow leads to difficult and painful walking, as the working muscles do not get adequate flow at times of demand. The intracellular enzymes in the substance of the heart muscle diminish in quantity and quality, affecting the quality of cardiac contraction.

With aging lining of the nose suffers reduction in blood supply. This leads to a dry and stuffy nose and crust formation. The reflexes of the nasal lining to changes in external temperature are less effective. The sinus cavities suffer stagnation of secretions and poor clearance. Drainage passages of the sinus into the nose become blocked. The nasal part of the pharynx suffers reduced blood supply and the lining of the cavity is not as healthy as before. Stagnation of secretions leads to sinus and upper respiratory infections. The capacity of the trachea and the rest of the respiratory tree to expand and contract is reduced. This affects the proper flow pattern of inhaled and exhaled air. The bronchi and bronchioles receive less blood, hence function less healthily. The cilia lining the respiratory tree does not clear toxins, debris, bacteria and other pathogenic material well. Reduction in the elasticity of lung tissue increases the work of breathing.

Number of pulmonary capillaries reduce in size and number, affecting ventilation and perfusion of gases. The elasticity of intercostal muscles and ribs is reduced, making breathing difficult. The diaphragm becomes rigid and inelastic, leading to difficulty in the proper up and down movement of the lungs and circulation of the energy drawn in. Clearance of toxins in the respiratory system is thus affected. The vital capacity of the lungs diminishes and the person is not as energetic as before. The cells not being able to secure a healthy supply of oxygen, cellular metabolic reactions are affected. The mitochondria need an adequate supply of oxygen.

With aging, atrophy of salivary glands leads to decreased salivation, dryness of the mouth and impaired digestion. Oral ulcers and inflammation of the tongue, with loss of taste, occur due to atrophy of the taste buds. Loss of teeth due to weakening of tissues and retraction of the gingiva is common. Swallowing is difficult because of weak pharyngeal muscles. Blood flow to all the organs reduces, to the detriment of their efficient functioning.

Reduction in the motility of the esophagus makes swallowing difficult and prolongs its peristaltic activity. The muscle layer of the stomach is not as efficient as before, and the action of churning food is weaker. The cells of the stomach atrophy, resulting in diminished acid outflow and poor appetite. Improper nutrition affects body weight. Secretion of the 'intrinsic factor', which is important for absorption of vitamin B_{12}, is affected. Iron absorption is also poor due to reduced acid output. This causes anaemia. As acid secretion is reduced, invasion of the stomach by pathogenic organisms leads to gastritis, bloating, belching and excessive wind formation with discomfort. Reflex responses of other glandular secretions to unloading of gastric contents into the duodenum is sluggish, with resultant indigestion and fat malabsorption.

Carbohydrate intolerance, with diminished ability to handle a glucose load, is due to an aging pancreas with loss of islet cells. The gall bladder begins to atrophy, impairing the excretion of bile, leading to fat emulsification with formation of gall stones. The amount of subcutaneous fat in the body reduces. Sensitivity of the body cells to insulin also decreases as one ages. The smooth muscles in the walls of the intestines become inelastic, causing retention of gases. The peristaltic capacity of the ileum and colon becomes weak. This hinders proper absorption of food and water, with reduction in assimilation. Elimination of waste matter is sluggish. The build up of colonic toxins increases the chances of colon cancer. The cells in the wall of the colon get dehydrated. This reduces the water content of waste matter, causing the passage of dry stools and consequent constipation.

Cellular function of the alimentary tract is affected due to poor blood supply. The flow of digestive juices decreases. The villous cells of the intestine suffer poor blood flow and lymphatic circulation, and hence absorption of nutrients is poor. Hardening of the arteries affects the blood flow to the gastrointestinal tract. An emergency condition, ischaemic necrosis of the wall of the intestine, can be caused. A diet poor in fibre and lack of exercise lead to diverticulosis, a condition where the walls of the intestine form sac-like dilatations.

Body metabolism is decreasing with aging. Due to poor physical activity, the metabolic rate slows down. This is aggravated by poor absorption of food. The hampering of circulation, respiration, nervine and glandular functions further affects metabolic activity. Efficient metabolic activity is an expression of inner energy.

Changes occurring in renal system with aging is shown up clearly. Blood flow into the filtration areas being reduced, cellular functioning is affected. The quality and quantity of urine outflow is altered. The organs start shrinking. Hardening of the renal arteries causes rise in blood pressure in the body, due to certain reflex chemical changes. The bladder wall suffers from poor tone and bladder capacity reduces. Stasis of urine is common, due to poor muscle function leading to urinary infections. The prostate enlarges, pressing on the urethra. Symptoms of outflow obstruction may be severe enough to require surgery. Aging of the female urinary tract is dealt with in the discussion of menopause, as the condition is linked to hormonal changes.

By aging the nervous system cannot regenerate as before and their efficiency is reduced. The delivery of nutrients and oxygen is reduced due to a weaker heart, which further affects the functioning of the brain. This sort of change occurs in all the divisions of the nervous system, resulting in their poor functioning. Increase in the build-up of toxic waste material in the interior of the neurons causes various diseases. The speed with which the nervous system reacts to physical and mental situations is affected. Hardening of the blood vessels causes cerebral ischaemia and sudden rupture and bleeding. The most common situation is when a person finishes a meal and suddenly insists that he or she has not eaten at all.

Poor functioning of brain causes lack of vitality throughout the body. The cerebellar cells atrophy, affecting balance and coordination. The regulatory centres in the cerebral cortex and medulla controlling cardiovascular, respiratory and endocrine functions become less effective. The lower centres in the spinal cord do not exercise adequate bladder and bowel control, resulting in uninhibited voiding and defecation. The centres in the spinal cord function less effectively. More time is taken to transmit and act on messages to and from the brain.

Aging causes reduced blood supply to the eye and retina. Night vision is hampered. The choroid becomes less vascular. The nerves supplying the iris become sluggish. The dilating and constricting capacity of the pupil is less effective. The cornea becomes less transparent due to a diminished flow of fluid in the tissues of the eye. Lipids are deposited on the edge of the cornea, causing a characteristic lining of the entire corneal curve, known as arcus senilis. Associated elevation of serum cholesterol is often present. The conjunctiva and sclera become dry as the tear gland is not as effective as before. Poor or total stoppage of tear secretions irritate the eye, with resultant inflammation and infection. Blood flow to the ear is reduced, resulting in nerve deafness. The balancing mechanism is also affected. This leads to diminished ability to adjust to postural imbalances and even normal activity. The nasal lining atrophies, reducing healthy olfactory capacity.

The glands are very important for optimum metabolic activity, one of the most important being the activity of the thyroid gland. Hypofunctioning is common in old age. Glandular function is important for many functions in the body: absorption, utilisation, enzyme actions and storage of absorbed material. The blood supply to the pituitary reduces, and the nervine connection with the hypothalamus is less effective. The pancreas does not perform as before. The adrenal glands are probably the most affected. The level of chemicals in the gland is lower, and the ability of the gland to react to acute situations is weaker.

As the endocrine system is also responsible for bone and muscle health, poor functioning of the glands affects them. Bone density is deficient, as is muscle mass. This is also related to poor dietary intake and lack of exercise. Decline in glandular functioning leads to overall decline in energy, enhanced susceptibility to infections, diminished physical drive and wasting of the body. Recovery from fatigue takes longer due to decreased capacity of the cells to respond to stimuli.

Muscles are very sensitive to usage or the lack of it and suffer deconditioning very rapidly, especially if the person has been in the habit of exercising regularly. The difference is more perceptible here. The enzymes available in the muscle cells also reduce, affecting contractile capacity. The connective tissues of the body become rigid and desiccated. This affects the resilience of the musculoskeletal system, causing greater mechanical load on the joints. Loss of flexibility in the joints results in arthritis.

Reduced water content in the discs makes for loss of resilience, decreases the height of the spinal column, causes rigidity of the associated structures and increased incidence of fractures of the bones.

Mineral content of the bone reduces due to poor nutrition and absorption, lack of exercise and, in women, menopause. The deposition of calcium in women's bones is an estrogen-dependent mechanism, and lack of this results in osteoporosis. Body movements are slower. Injuries take time to heal due to reduced vascularity of the tissues. Increased stiffness in joints can cause periarthritis of the shoulder and osteoarthritis of the finger, spine, knee and shoulder joints. Fractures of the hip are common. General body usage is more tiring than before and recuperating takes time. Menopausal woman suffers more from musculoskeletal disorders.

There is no medicine that can prevent all these systems from failing in old age. Exercise and a healthy diet are the only answers. A lifestyle which is based on these two essentials greatly precludes the risk of certain kinds of cancer. Today medicine has found out that age is no bar to improving ones's exercise capacity which, in turn, improves health. There are a variety of exercises. The more severe the exercise, the more the level of free radicals produced. During exercise, oxidative reactions increase and damage to tissue is bound to occur. Over-exercising the body produces more radicals and under-exercising fails to remove the toxins. The optimum amount of exercise enhances the defence systems of cells which remove free radicals.

When a radical reacts with an unsaturated fatty acid of the cell structure, a new radical is formed. In the presence of oxygen this new radical initiates a process known as lipid peroxidation of cell membranes, resulting in cellular swelling and tissue inflammation. When lipid peroxides split, the hydrocarbons pentane and ethane are formed. The levels of gases increase with heavy exercise. Now, with yoga, the process of exercise is totally different. The process is light and energising, unlike endurance exercises; moreover, asanas help remove cellular toxins. Yoga, being a steady and slow system, does not result in free radicals being formed as fast as they are removed, as in other exercises.

Asanas and pranayama induce cellular quietening, thus inducing a state of hibernation. Hence, free radicals are removed by the massaging action of asanas and optimum formation of radicals is maintained throughout the practice session without irritation. According to yoga, the mind controls the production of free radicals, both at rest and during exercise. If there is excessive stress of the mind, the body suffers. If the mind is not used, the body still suffers stagnation of radicals. A healthy mind optimises free radical production and removal. In other systems the mind is exhausted and strained. One of the key points in yoga is that the asanas are practised with proper alignment and centring. There is a precise method and only one optimum way in which the right effect is given to the internal organs.

In yoga, the liver or spleen may be directly massaged, the brain directly rinsed with blood, all at no expense to any other parameter. Other exercises act as irritative systems, by increasing pulse rate and blood pressure. At this expense, circulation is thought to be improved. During exercise, blood is shunted away from the skin and certain other areas to nourish the vital organs and the muscles. It might be dangerous for the cardiac patient to jog, as the heart can be irritated; but in yoga, there is no irritation as the heart can be rested in the asanas, yet coronary flow improved without strain.

Yoga prevents atherosclerosis, maintaining the blood flow by auto-massage and preventing deposits being formed in the blood vessels. Moreover, blood is channelised to the organs in a very controlled way. Energy levels are very high in a body in which circulation of body fluids is well maintained, blood flow to the vital organs well preserved, and the intake of oxygen equal to that of a man in his twenties. For a normal person, the capacity to maintain cerebral perfusion in different postures from sitting to lying down is known as orthostatic tolerance. Athletes, used to high intensity training, where the volume of blood increases several times and the nerves are set to a higher level of stimulation, were found lacking in this capacity. Such changes do not happen to the yogic practitioner.

Yoga prevents changes in skeletal, renal, hepatic, neurological, cardiac and pulmonary systems by various mechanisms. The asanas act by rinsing organs with blood. This improves their cellular functions and maintains the elasticity of all the tissues. Pranayama prevents atmospheric damage to the cardiac system, as it washes away accumulated toxins in the blood.

In yoga, preferential shunting of blood is possible. The circulation to the skin is not at all reduced as in endurance exercises. On the contrary, blood flow to the skin is enhanced due to the massaging effect of the asanas. The shunting of blood in other exercises is involuntary, whereas in yoga one can shunt blood to any area consciously, as the geometric shapes of the asanas vary. The lungs get exhausted in endurance training. The mitochondria are flogged to the maximum with respect to their cellular power and respiratory functions. The strong lung capacity of an athlete is achieved by hard and forceful usage which is not conducive to preserving health. One can maintain the health of the lungs by the practice of back bends which are tougher than a running bout.

Abdominal organs are shaken to the maximum in the process of running. A forceful method is used as the pace of organ functioning is raised. The mechanical effect of the asanas—squeezing, rinsing, flushing, pressurising, etc.,—preserve cellular integrity very well. The delivery of nutrients is enhanced and, there is no wastage of reserves. The asanas promote blood flow to the oral cavity and maintain all the organs in the cavity.

Yoga has certain restful postures that re-energise the body under such conditions. This is the greatest advantage of yoga—an exercise which is useful during fatigue. The nerves are not exhausted in yogic practice. Though exercise improves energy levels by boosting the nervine functions, it is possible to achieve the same effect without exhaustion. In the long run, soft and gentle methods are more conducive to health. The endocrine glands are the keys to healthy energy levels. The hormones are not wasted in the practice of asanas. In endurance exercise, the glands get exhausted. Endurance training results in heavy excretion of cellular waste products and wastage of body protein which strains the kidneys.

In everyday life the usage of nerves is so erratic and exaggerated that, at the end of the day, we have very little energy left. Sleep gives rest to the cells of the body. Yoga is like sleep, where the sympathetic tone of the body falls, as asanas are maintained in a very silent and still manner without effort. The mind is kept very quiet for several hours at a stretch and profound relaxation occurs in both body and mind. The nerves thus recover very fast. One feels soothed after a prolonged practice of asanas because of rest to the sympathetic system which brings the body temperature to a lower level.

Force of gravity acts on the human body and tires it by constantly exerting traction on the nerves, veins and arteries. Yoga has poses that reverse the effects of this gravitational force so that lightness is imparted to the body. An organ that feels light is a healthy organ. Due to inverted asanas, aging in the central nervous system is avoided. This is due to the energisation of certain important nerve centres in the cerebral cortex and the brain stem. Muscle biopsy studied from persons who have trained by other exercises shows change in cellular architecture.

In yoga, cellular structure does not undergo any change as the nature of stimulus is different and hence there is no need for the body to adapt. The muscles are often damaged in endurance training. The chemical reserves are often altered. Depletion of glycogen is possible. In yoga such changes do not happen.

In yoga there is no pile-driver action, but a steady strain where a single or a group of muscles may be contracting and stretching at the same time. This combined action on a single muscle is unique to yoga. Hence yoga can be classified neither as isometric nor as isotonic. This action feeds the bone with healthy blood for the marrow. Where all other systems build up the bone in a convex shape, yoga does not cause hypertrophy. The bones remain strong yet slender in appearance. Physiologically, there is no need for the bones and muscles to hypertrophy for efficient function.

According to yoga, a muscle is healthy if its blood supply is maintained and it is mechanically sound. For a woman in menopause, the side effects of flushing, sudden sweats, palpitations, bone pain, fatigue, can all be debilitating. Asanas and pranayama help regulate the actions of the autonomic nervous system through which many side effects of menopause are mediated. It has been shown that exercise is of great value to the menopausal woman, preventing osteoporosis and other mechanical changes.

Effect of exercise on the immune system is a field of intense research. Exercise helps better functioning of the immune cells. In yoga, regional immunity can be improved because the blood can be flushed into any area. This increases the concentration of immunity cells in those areas. In patients suffering from recurrent sore throats, the practice of sarvangasana greatly reduces the frequency of infections. Immunity is also improved by the destressing of the body and mind. It is well known that under stress the functioning of the immune system is affected. We know the skeletal movements of extension, flexion, rotation and so on. Every organ has to be treated in this way. This is known as healthy exercise. Yoga is an organic movement and not a physical one at all.

If there is pain on one side while doing yoga, analyse the side that has the pain, analyse the side that has no pain, then try to do the same good movement on the affected side. This requires great sensitivity. The movement in yoga has to coordinate the skin, muscles, joints and inner organs, all in a single movement of the asana to obtain correct effects. This is integrated yogic practice, which has to be done mathematically and geometrically. The asanas have to be practised with lightness and vigour and not in a heavy, lethargic manner.

There is no age bar to the practice of yoga. Any person who is not lethargic in the pursuit of different forms of yoga attains *siddhi* through practice, be he young, old or even very old sickly or weak. The props help in the execution of the poses. Other exercises may be contraindicated for a patient with a cardiac problem, or hypertension, or some other ailment. But yoga can always be practised, with asanas specified for the medical problem.

REFERENCES

Edwards, Sally, *Sally Edwards' Heart Zone Training: Exercise Smart, Stay Fit, And Live Longer*, Holbrook, MA: Adams Publishing, 1996.

Dr.Krishna Raman, *A Matter of Health: Intergration of Yoga and Western Meidcine to Prevention and Care*, 1998, Eastwest Books, Madras.

On The Run: Exercise And Fitness For Busy People, Waitz, Grete Paperback ISBN: 1579542530.

Scott K. Powers Stephen L. Dodd, *Total Fitness: Exercise, Nutrition, and Wellness*, 1999.

Sharon A. Plowman Denise L. Smith, *Exercise Physiology: For Health, Fitness and Performance*, 1997.

Terry J. Housh Ph.D. Dona J. Housh Ph.D., *Introduction to Exercise Science*, 2000

Thomas D. Fahey Ed.D., *Super Fitness for Sports, Conditioning, and Health*, 2000.

8

Population Health: The Millennium Vision

The scientific developments in medicine are one of the wonders of the twentieth century, with advances in diagnostic technology, surgery, and pharmaceuticals that no one would have predicted several decades ago. New treatments for cancer and for heart disease have contributed to the quantifiable increased life expectancy we now enjoy. Other examples of clinical interventions of great benefit are hip replacements that provide improved quality of life in elderly patients and the chemical treatment of depression. Other progresses are expected from advances in new pharmaceuticals, genetic engineering, non-invasive therapies, and behavioural medicine, in the future.

The challenge now in purchasing population health, in an era of limited resources, is to move toward that optimal balance of resource allocation across the known determinants of health that will produce the greatest improvement for the most people with the resources available. Many discussions of the determinants of health have difficulty avoiding a tone that is critical of medical care; this understandably offends health professionals and confuses patients who have benefited from medical care. It often appears that one has to take one side or the other: that of total reliance on and respect for medical care or; alternatively, questioning the value of any scientific or medical intervention.

It would be hard to discount the financial and professional power of physicians and the medical industry, which provides a target for these criticisms. In fact, it is undoubtedly the wonders of modern medicine that are responsible for the dominant public view that medical care is the only or the predominant contributor to health. The parallel truth is that there is a less well recognised but large and growing body of evidence supporting the independent contributions of factors other than medical care in the health of populations.

People become sick for a variety of unspecified reasons and present themselves to the health care system for care and cure. The health care system is both a thermostat and furnace, with the response to colder temperatures (more disease) being to turn up the heat (more health care). In this view of the world, health policy is identical to health care policy, with no other factors or determinants recognised. Recall that disease is distinct from both health and function as well as from well-being. Disease is the dysfunction identified and treated by the medical care system, while the concept of health and function explains the manner in which symptoms and conditions are experienced by the individual.

The concept of well-being is a higher order function, that of total life satisfaction, which is broader than that of health and function. In addition to health care, other factors impact on both disease and health and on function. It identifies the broad categories of genetic endowment, the physical environment, and the social environment as not only influencing disease but also as playing a role in the individual response to both disease and to health and function.

A major evidence for the role of non-medical factors in population health is the persistent finding that higher levels of socio-economic status are directly associated with lower levels of mortality and morbidity. This has been termed the socioeconomic gradient in health status. Socio-economic status is a concept that generally includes such factors as education, income, and social/occupational class; these are obviously interrelated factors, and care must be taken when attempting to explain their independent impact on health. The most important work in understanding this relationship is that of the British social epidemiologist Michael Marmot and his colleagues. Their initial findings came from a unique data set called the *Whitehall Survey*, which followed more than 10,000 British civil servants over more than two decades. These middle-aged male employees were grouped into four occupational classifications according to hierarchy and status: administrative, professional-executive, clerical, and others.

The striking initial findings were that age-adjusted mortality rates were three and one-half times higher in the lowest status manual grade than in the highest administrative grade, and that there was a gradient in mortality from the lowest to the highest. Very striking is the finding that the mortality gradient still remained when traditional risk factors were taken into account. Lower status employees have higher levels of risk factors such as smoking, high blood pressure, and high cholesterol but that most of the differences in mortality are unexplained by these risk factors. In addition, historical data in England show that a similar gradient has persisted over most of the years since 1911 when the data were first collected.

All these persons were employed in government civil service jobs, and so these differences cannot be explained by poverty or extreme deprivation. Recent evidence is beginning to shed light on which aspects of occupational hierarchy are related to the risk of mortality, with level of control over job function emerging as important.

Education has a major role in maintaining health status and mortality for some time, particularly in developing countries. The relationship between maternal literacy and child mortality has been clearly established. Initially this was thought to operate through the increased economic status that greater literacy brings, but recent studies have isolated the independent effect of literacy and schooling from income levels.

A 1985 United Nations study of 15 developing countries indicated that the effect of an additional year of mother's schooling resulted in a 3.4 per cent reduction in mortality; this impact was greater than the sum of doubling income, piped water, and toilets as well as moving from agricultural to white collar work. In the United States, in 1973 Kitagawa and Hauser demonstrated a graded relationship between education and mortality, with significantly lower levels of mortality in 1960 for those with college education than for those with less than high school levels.

A recent study in the United States by Pappas and his colleagues reanalysed the data of Kitagawa and Hauser from 1960 and extended it to 1986. They showed that mortality rates were lower but that decreases in mortality were greatest in the more educated groups. This indicates not only that the gradient persists but that the inequality in mortality in relation to educational level has increased in each subgroup of the population over the 26 years studied; for African American and white men it doubled, and it grew 30 percent for African American women and 23 per cent for white women. Another study, by Guralnik and colleagues, compared whites and African Americans in 1987 in the North Carolina Piedmont area with regard to active life expectancy. Mortality differences between older African Americans and whites were eliminated when adjusting for educational level between the racial groups; higher educational attainment was related to a marked advantage in all race-gender subgroups. The increase ranged from 2.5 to 4.6 years of life expectancy and from 2.4 to 3.9 years of active (disability-free) life expectancy.

Increasing the likelihood that a person will attain a high level of education not only may be advantageous for that person's young and middle years as a wage earner but also may be a valuable investment in increasing his or her years of active, non-disabled life after retirement. The association of higher education level with longer and healthier life does not explain the mechanism for the relationship. Speculation has centred on the impact that knowledge has on productivity and income, on more appropriate utilisation of health services, on healthier lifestyles (e.g., with regard to alcohol consumption, smoking, driving), and on community cohesion.

Smoking behaviour partially explains the impact of education on mortality for middle-aged and older persons and was found to be primarily responsible for the impact of educational levels on low-birth-weight babies. The distinguished economist Victor Fuchs has observed that education helps individuals make better use of available medical care resources, as well as helping them better appreciate the importance of making current health investments (i.e., stopping smoking) for future benefit.

There might be a relationship between income and health status. Many studies, particularly of developing countries, have shown such results, especially at the low end of the income scale. Early studies documented relationships between lack of social integration and suicide, tuberculosis, accidents, and schizophrenia; in addition, married persons have lower age adjusted mortality rates from all causes than unmarried persons. In these early studies, however, it was not clear if poor health caused the poor relationships or vice versa. The 1970s saw a great expansion of research in this field, driven by interest in stress and psychosocial relationships in death and disease.

In 1979, Berkman and Syme reported on a prospective survey in Alameda County, California, that overcame some of the limitations of previous research. They examined the impact on mortality of a social network index comprising four factors: marriage, contacts with family and friends, church membership, and other formal and informal group affiliations. They found that persons low on the index were twice as likely to die as those high on the index, after controlling for other factors such as physical health, socio-economic status, smoking, alcohol consumption, obesity, and use of preventive services.

Dressler has examined the reasons for higher levels of hypertension in African Americans and finds that darker skin colour is associated with higher blood pressure levels, independent of socio-economic variables. He and others provide beginning evidence that suggests that frustrating social interactions and colour-based barriers, including greater unemployment, family instability, and criminal victimisation, can produce stress that has other pathophysiologic effects such as poor pregnancy outcomes, diabetes, and even cancer and heart disease.

There are racial differences in mortality and use of services among Medicare beneficiaries. Feagin has observed that many African Americans experience more than isolated incidents of discrimination, including repeated blatant acts of violence, verbal harassment, and physical attack combined with subtle and covert slights, accumulated over months, years and lifetimes, which have an impact far more than the sum of individual instances.

Social scientists have been examining the reasons for problems that communities and nations have in mutual cooperation; failures of such cooperation and joint action certainly contribute to many of our recognised social problems in areas such as public education, inner city crime, and environmental global warming. In such situations, everyone would be better off if there were an increased degree of cooperation. Robert Putnam, a sociologist at Harvard, and his colleagues developed the concept of social capital while trying to explain the successes and failures of some regional governments in Italy since 1970. Those that failed were characterised by inefficiency, lethargy, and corruption, while others were remarkably successful in economic development, community programmes, environmental standards, and support for families.

The best predictor of effectiveness was what they called strong traditions of civic engagement, such as voter turnout, newspaper readership, membership in choral societies and literary clubs, and participation in civic organisations and soccer teams. They termed this factor social capital and described it in an analogous fashion to physical and human capital, as an economic factor that enhances individual productivity. The term refers to features of social organisation such as networks, norms, and trust that facilitate coordination and cooperation for mutual benefit. While the work of Putnam and his colleagues does not focus on health *per se*, they note that there have been similar studies that link neighbourhood characteristics with teen pregnancy rates in both African Americans and whites, controlling for individual differences; similar factors have been related to coronary artery disease mortality. This is a broader context for the influence of socio-economic factors, both for health status and for well-being.

Indeed, some economists such as Amaryta Sen argue that traditional neoclassical economics with its primary focus on individual economic improvement is limited in explaining individual and community decisions to forgo short-run economic gain for longer benefit to the community or society.

Although the social determinants of health are not as widely appreciated as medical or biologic ones, the evidence presented in the previous sections is quite compelling. But how do such factors impact on length and quality of life, which are biologic in the final effect? Even though there is much in medicine regarding causation that is not certain, basic mechanisms such as cholesterol plaques plugging arteries, cigarette tar causing lung cells to become cancerous, and infectious agents such as viruses destroying certain cell types are generally understood.

Most of the evidence on the role of stress comes from animal studies that try to make the link between the socioeconomic environment and individual biology. While it is beyond the scope of this chapter to cover this evidence in great detail, a few examples are helpful. It has long been understood that the body has endocrine mechanisms that respond to stressful situations by increasing the output of certain hormones such as adrenaline. This allows us to respond appropriately in times of danger. But there is also evidence that constant stress may eventually result in a lowered capacity of response.

In an interesting work, Sapolsky has shown that the mechanism in rats that reduces stress hormone production becomes less effective over time and therefore produces a vicious cycle in which prolonged exposure to stress produces increasing vulnerability to it, accelerating the aging process. In addition, he has found in baboons in Kenya that lower status baboons are less able to turn off the hormone responses to stress and therefore suffer the biologic consequences of higher stress levels. This finding suggests possible connections to the evidence linking job status with mortality in British civil servants.

All job classes have higher blood pressure at work than at home, but the blood pressure of those in higher job classifications drops more at home than that of those in lower grades, suggesting that the former are able to turn off the stress response more effectively. In other studies in monkeys designed to test coronary artery response to high cholesterol diets, the degree of artery narrowing was four times greater in low status monkeys than in the high status groups. While the precise biological mechanisms for these effects are not fully known, they seem to lie in the interconnected pathways between hormones and the immune system; indeed an entire new area of research has been labelled psycho-neuro-immunology.

Enough evidence has already been accumulated to suggest possible biologic pathways for the impact of socio-economic conditions on health; this should stimulate much more research in this field, as well as blunting the criticism of those who assert that such relationships cannot be important because a feasible mechanism of effect has not been discovered. It is important in this context to pay special attention to issues in child development, because they influence the entire lifespan. It is well understood that early influences can have profound effects on child development at very basic neurological and brain development levels, and more evidence is accumulating as to how these influences play out over the life course.

The impact of cultural factors was implicitly assumed to operate at the individual level. But it is also possible that characteristics of the entire society or culture modify the response to various factors. A comparative study of Britain and Sweden found similar trends in occupational grade and health, but the gradient was much less pronounced. Although socio-economic factors are external to the organism, genetic determinants are deeply embedded within cells and nucleic acid. Health results from interactions between individuals and their social and physical environments. The individual has genes that cannot adapt to ordinary environments. A hostile environment overwhelms the genetic adaptive capacity. A combination of environmental insult and genetic predisposition results in disease.

At one extreme there are individuals who have a genetically determined metabolism that causes symptoms even when cholesterol levels in diets are normal. The other extreme is those whose metabolism of cholesterol is intact but whose very heavy cholesterol intake overwhelms normal metabolic mechanisms. If dietary cholesterol is low in the culture or sub-population, the percentage of cases from genetic metabolic factors will necessarily be greater. Due to of such interactions, in addition to the way mortality is classified, it is not possible to quantify precisely the contribution of genetic factors to death and disease.

Many failed pregnancies are the result of genetic abnormalities and chromosome defects. Five per cent of individuals have a disease of genetic origin significant enough to require treatment before age 25. Infant mortality is now one-third from genetic causes. Over age 25, more than 60 per cent of diseases of late onset may have genetics as one contributing factor.

Classically Mendelian genetic disorders, which reduce the lifespan and cause psychological handicaps, are primarily found in early life, with 90 per cent appearing by the end of puberty. In later life, genetic variability of populations decreases as those with the least adaptive genes die, leaving most of the remaining elderly with non-genetic disease. The field of genetic epidemiology is concerned with the reasons diseases cluster in families and ethnic groups, and it tries to determine whether the clustering is caused by common environmental exposure, biologically inherited susceptibility, and/or culturally inherited risk factors.

Using creative methods such as twin studies, adoption studies, and migration studies, some of these genetic and environmental factors can be separated. Hereditary factors have been identified for schizophrenia, alcoholism, and high blood pressure; examples of genetic factors are found in sickle cell anaemia, Down's syndrome, and susceptibility to malaria. There is significant controversy about whether or what degree intervention in the genetic make-up of individuals and populations would be an effective or acceptable strategy for increasing population health.

The excitement of the Human Genome Project and the initial experiments in laboratory animals raise the possibility that altering the frequency of some genes in individuals or populations would contribute to future population health improvement. But there are several lines of caution in placing major emphasis on this approach. The first is that the genetic reservoir of variation is one way that the species evolves and deals with future environmental change. Tampering with this in an attempt to create genetic endowments that are ideal is risky, if not fraught with ethical considerations.

In addition, most genetic disorders are complex multi-gene interactions, which we are far from being able to manipulate in humans. Finally, the impact on mortality and morbidity is very often the result of interactions between host susceptibility and environmental influences, including lifestyle. For many genetic diseases, the environmental factors may be quicker and less costly to change.

Efforts directed toward environmental protection and restoration have been a major social movement of the late twentieth century, drawing the attention of people concerned about the future of the world in which they live. The field of environmental health is a broad one, dealing both with the impact of the environment on people and that of people on the environment. Components include air, water, and food quality, waste disposal, rodents and insects, injury control, radiation, workplace safety, and issues concerning energy sources and use. Both short- and long-term considerations such as global warming and acid rain are encompassed. With regard to health outcomes, the Centres for Disease Control and Prevention have estimated a range of 57,000 to 108,000 deaths in 1990 that could be attributed to what they term toxic ugents. These pose threats as occupational hazards, environmental pollutants, contaminants of food and water supplies, and components of commercial products. These agents are known to have an impact on all organ systems, including the heart, lungs, liver, kidneys, bladder, and the nervous system.

The morbidity of such toxic exposure is more difficult to measure but is perhaps more important than mortality. For example, lead poisoning is rarely fatal, but the neurologic and mental damage to the more than 230,000 children having high blood lead levels is certainly significant. Asthma kills about 5,000 people per year but also contributes significantly to absence from school and work; for asthma a major risk factor or trigger is air pollution as well as cockroaches in the living environment.

Reproductive outcomes are impacted by eating contaminated fish. We are all aware of disease and morbidity caused by food impurity, by water contamination, and by workplace injury. Ostro showed that a 10 per cent increase in the total suspended particles in urban air samples resulted in a

4.5 per cent increase in the number of workdays lost, and Mullahy and Portney were able to show that increased cigarette consumption was about 2.5 times more important in causing restricted activity than increases in ozone concentration.

There is evidence that environmental quality varies by race and income, with lower socio-economic groups having higher exposure to toxic wastes and air pollution. With current efforts for environmental cleanup gaining public attention, perhaps it is possible to reduce vigilance in this area. However, more subtle environmental sentinels in wildlife, particularly regarding hormonal changes, are cause for concern. Broader environmental issues such as ozone depletion and global warming may have health and social consequences that are not yet fully appreciated. The field of environmental health has also provided us with some of the best analytic methods regarding exposure and risk and long-run cost benefit analysis.

Healthy People 2000, the 1990 statement of health goals for the nation, included eight behaviours that required improvement for health promotion:

a) physical activity and fitness;
b) awareness of nutrition and the hazards of tobacco, alcohol, and other drugs;
c) family planning;
d) dentificated treatment of mental health and emotional disorders;
e) avoidance of violent and abusive behaviour; and
f) establishment of community-based education programmes.

A 1995 report on mid-decade progress on these goals noted substantial reduction in adult tobacco use, alcohol-related automobile deaths and a modest improvement in diet but no reductions in sedentary lifestyle or weight. Knowles listed several reasons in 1977. They include:

a) the denial of death coupled with demand for instant gratification;
b) the belief that science and technology will conquer nature;
c) chronic depression causing disinterest or inactivity; and
d) the focus of medicine and physicians on cure rather than prevention.

Such factors are supported by current anecdotal information that the availability of new AIDS protease inhibitor drugs has resulted in an increase of unsafe sex practices. Some health behaviourists and public health educators are beginning to think much more broadly about such challenges, applying strategies of social marketing to sophisticated public health communication. This entails strategies such as targeting messages to homogeneous audiences, presenting information about risks from behavioural choices, developing mass media advocacy, building information strategies into entertainment programming, and encouraging the use of computer interactive patient education programmes for sensitive topics like sexual behaviour.

Providing consumers with information and guidelines about self-care and increasing their confidence about making medical decisions can be effective; in addition, health promotion in the workplace has been shown to reduce absenteeism and medical care expenditures. In the area of prevention and health promotion, it is not the lack of scientific knowledge that limits us, but our ability to apply existing knowledge. This is difficult, because in many cases we are dealing with fundamental issues of values, beliefs, culture, and individual rights.

Health improvement is not an individual responsibility alone. Certain aspects are a social responsibility, and the individual cannot solely be blamed for the poor health of the population. There are, for example, strong economic interests such as the tobacco industry that counter the efforts of health promotion. In addition, there are segments of society, many of low education and income, whose lives are desperate and for whom such imperatives such as good nutrition are remote or economically impossible. For these reasons there is societal as well as individual responsibility for health behaviour change, and a combined strategy is required if optimal progress in improving population health outcomes is to be achieved.

The Institute of Medicine (IOM) defined the mission of public health as fulfilling society's interest in assuring conditions in which people can be healthy. It does this by encouraging action of others in public and private sectors, by regulation requiring action, and by providing direct services. Afifi and Breslow define the core disciplines of public health as epidemiology, biostatistics, personal health services, health behaviour, and environmental health and define public health practice as those actions that are directed to the assessment of health and disease in the population, the formulation of policies for dealing with such problems, and the assurance of environmental, behavioural, and medical services designed to accelerate favourable health trends and reduce the unfavourable.

During the health reform debate in 1993 and 1994, the expectation of universal coverage for personal health services led to active discussion of reinventing public health in a post-universal coverage world, since this critical safety net personal health provider role to the uninsured and geographically isolated would have been assumed by the proposed alliances and plans.

Since universal coverage remains an unfilled priority, the role of public health as a critical provider of last resort remains. But for the majority of insured Americans, almost all of their personal care is provided outside of the traditional state and local public health systems, causing definitional confusion since the role that medical care plays in health status is then not primarily in the public sector.

Certainly public health departments have critical core population based roles in environmental services and protection. Given their expertise in community prevention activities, they also have essential roles for public education, behaviour change, and outreach services to high-risk populations. If a fundamental role is the assurance of healthy conditions, then an expanding core function of public health agencies has to be in the data collection or monitoring function for measuring population health improvement. If public health is to reinvent its role, the weakened system needs to be strengthened. Distinct policies are needed to strengthen the infrastructure for delivering population-based services at the state and local levels and to encourage the public and personal health care systems to work constructively together.

The public health system is uniquely qualified to provide population-based community health services. However without expanding health insurance coverage, the public health system will not be able to move away from providing medical care to the indigent and uninsured and the infrastructure will continue to deteriorate.

Changes in life expectancy will occur in the long run, whether they are the result of medical or non-medical factors. The result is that future cohorts will have greater (or less) future life expectancy than previous cohorts of similar age. Even if changes in life expectancy were the result of prevention in the medical care system such as lowering cholesterol levels, the resulting improvement would be detected only in future years.

Furthermore, morbidity is likely to be more amenable to intervention in the short run (e.g., hip replacement or treatment of depression) than mortality. In some cases, interventions might have impact on both life expectancy and morbidity (e.g., prenatal care and social support reducing low-birth-weight babies or a drug with short-term benefit and long-term side effects) and therefore would need to be measured in both the short run and the long run.

MEASURING HEALTH OUTCOMES

The population-based interventions of public health such as community health education and fluoridation of water are included, but much relevance is done in both the non-profit and for-profit private sectors. Health promotion and disease prevention as well as primary care are critical components, but many aspects of health improvement come from diagnosis and treatment in secondary and tertiary care as well. The first step is to distinguish between the concepts of health and population health.

The idea of health and function is defined from the perspective of the individual and family and is concerned with the impact of disease on the physical, mental, social, and occupational functions of people's lives. The concept of well-being transcends health policy alone and becomes a major objective of all human activity.

The population health perspective proposed here adopts the intermediate one of health and function as its basis, incorporating the expanded idea of maximising function in a number of domains. Such a framework requires an operational measure of population health that goes beyond quantity of life (mortality) to add extra dimensions. In other words, the goal is to purchase not only life years but life years at some level of quality.

The measurement of status of health has been of increasing concern to researchers and policymakers over the past several decades. An appropriate aggregate measure of health and function might be health adjusted life expectancy (HALE), which combines the length and quality of life into an estimate of the number of years that can be expected in a specified state of health: an international organisation fostering these concepts called the Network on Health Expectancy has been formed. Following this approach, measures like disability adjusted life years (DALYs), quality adjusted life years (QALYs), and years of healthy life (YHLs), are specific ways of measuring the generic HALE concept.

The sum of the health of individuals is, of course, equal to that of the population under consideration. However, this is too narrow a concept because it lulls us into thinking that improving health outcomes can be accomplished only by focusing on individual medical care interventions, which is still the dominant model operating today.

Population health goes beyond public health or population based interventions to include all aspects of medical care that are effective in improving individual health and function. But a population health framework adds two additional considerations beyond the sum of individual health adjusted life expectancy.

The first is a broad understanding of the determinants of health or HALE. In addition to the contributions made through medical care to individuals, progress in HALE also comes from improvements in socio-economic status through increased levels of education and income and from preventive services at a group or population level as well from investments in other sectors such as social services, genetics, and the environment. While this does not change the definition of total population health adjusted life expectancy, it requires a broader perspective than simply providing medical care to individuals.

Most of these non-medical interventions, such as public health education and efforts to improve the environment, are introduced at the community or social level but have direct or indirect impact on the health of individuals; good examples for thinking about this are the reduction of harmful contaminants in air or water, reducing crime and violence, and public advertising campaigns regarding smoking or sexually transmitted diseases (STDs).

If resources were not an issue, then any individual investment in medical care or other health determinants might be appropriate, even if it was very costly, was of questionable effectiveness, or was clearly ineffective but desired by the individual.

But given that health care is financed to a considerable degree with public funds and that employer and individual cash outlays are constrained as well, it is necessary to look at the most cost-effective means of getting value in terms of health outcomes. This will mean that expenditures on some individuals or on alternative determinants of health will have a much higher return than others in terms of the health adjusted life expectancy of the entire population. Making such resource allocation decisions is difficult and has distributional considerations.

Such allocation decisions are being made now, some explicitly and some implicitly. The population health perspective requires that purchasers, providers, and society consider the health of all individuals in addition to the health of particular individuals. This idea is summarised by the statement by Evans and Stoddart that a society that spends so much on health care that it cannot or will not spend adequately on other health-enhancing activities may actually be reducing the health of its population.

In a world where resources are limited, spending a large amount on one health determinant such as medical care, leaving fewer resources to invest in another area, such as the environment or education could negatively affect the health not only of individuals but of the whole population. Since purchasing population health requires a quantifiable measure for financial incentives, for this purpose population health is defined as the aggregate health outcome of health adjusted life expectancy of a group of individuals, in an economic framework that balances the relative marginal return from the multiple determinants of health.

Adopting a HALE framework for the definition of population health requires some concrete, operational measure of HALE that can be used for an accurate assessment of baseline health outcomes as well as any change from the baseline. Such a measure or measures must possess at least the following characteristics:

a) scientific credibility from a theoretical perspective,
b) unambiguous definition,

c) availability of appropriate data, and

d) validity for differentiating between various populations.

Mortality

While health-related quality of life adjustments occupy much of the current research attention in this field, mortality remains a critical and, perhaps, the ultimate health outcome.

There are several ways to measure life years or mortality using tools developed by demographers:

a) *Crude death rate*: The crude death rate expressed as deaths per 100,000 population. This statistic is available in most countries and is reported according to a standard set of international cause-of-death categories. The crude death rate is not usually used, since there are fundamental biologic differences in death rates by age and by gender. Therefore, if one population has more old persons or more males, its crude death rate would naturally be higher than one with fewer such persons.

b) *Age-adjusted death rates*: The most widely used corrected mortality rate is age adjusted death rate, or standardised mortality rate (SMR). This standardisation process essentially uses age-specific death rates for an entire population or a hypothetical standard one and creates a comparable age-adjusted death rate for the two populations as if their age distributions were similar. Because deaths are usually reported by cause, it is also useful to examine age-adjusted cause-specific death rates in order to analyse the diseases responsible for different death rates.

   Overall death rates have declined from 841 to 520 (per 100,000) over the 40 years, with major decreases in deaths resulting from heart disease, cerebrovascular causes (strokes), and pneumonia/influenza. Rates from some specific causes such as lung cancer, homicide, and, of course, AIDS have increased, both absolutely and as a percentage of the lower total.

c) *Life expectancy*: Life expectancy, or the years of life remaining for a population or age group is the number derived from demographic life tables and refers to the expected number of years that persons reaching a certain age will live. This needs to be presented at least for each gender, given the biologic differences in death rates between males and females.

d) *Infant mortality*: Infant mortality is defined not in relation to overall population but as the number of deaths under one year of age per 1,000 live births in the same year.

The World Bank has used the concept of time lost to premature death, in which age adjusted death rates are compared to an international standard of achievement; others have occasionally made comparisons with what biologists might estimate maximum or ideal life expectancy to be. Sometimes premature death rate estimates are reported as age adjusted death rates before age 65. In 1996 when Senator Nancy Kassebaum requested that the US General Accounting Office identify the best way to determine the relative health needs of states, in order to have a way to allocate the funds in a new $1.1 billion public health block grant programme, the premature mortality measure was identified as the single best proxy for reflecting differences in the health status of states' populations.

Some measure of mortality needs to form the basis of a new outcome purchasing standard, since there is no quality of life without life itself. Estimating the life expectancy of sub-populations, either by geographic location or by membership in a specific health plan, is complicated by changes in plan membership as well as by the uncertainty of future mortality rates for each age group, given the reductions that have already occurred over time.

In addition, sub-populations may have additional biological or demographic characteristics that result in different distributions of life expectancy within the group. These heterogeneities clearly need to be recognised and dealt with when designing measurement standards for provider payment for purchasing population health.

There is more to health than simply years of life. In addition, because mortality is a relatively infrequent event, it causes statistical measurement problems in small populations. Advances beyond mortality have been made possible through new methods for assessing the quality of life in specific disease states and for general health status. A considerable body of evidence has been accumulated regarding the validity and reliability of various approaches, drawing on concepts from psychology, sociology, economics, and operations research.

Patrick and Bergner have categorised the domains of quality of life into relatively objective dimensions of impairment, including symptoms, physical function, psycho-logical function, and social function; the more subjective dimen-sions of perceptions, including general health perceptions and satisfactions; and the domain of opportunity, which includes concepts of disadvantage and resilience. In addition, they make the point that most research has focused on negative aspects of health and therefore considers health improvement to be a reduction in illness or health related dysfunction and/or lengthening of life.

It is important to identify positive enhancements in relatively well individuals such as increased energy, stamina, feeling of well-being, resilience, and productivity, even if longevity and morbidity are unaffected. There is often definitional ambiguity about the concept of quality of life and the components or boundaries of morbidity and disability. People can exit from morbidity and disability by recovery, remission, or death; people can only move from disability to morbidity. These illustrative survival curves indicate the percentage of persons remaining alive, disabled, or reporting morbidity at each age.

Morbidity

Morbidity data are generally concerned with the incidence and prevalence of specific medical conditions in the population. There has recently been active discussion about the impact of increasing life expectancy on morbidity. In the 1980s, survey data from the previous decade revealed increasing numbers of chronic conditions and activity limitations among older persons, which were interpreted to reflect increased morbidity resulting from longer life and were termed the failure of success. Others reviewed these trends and suggested that the reported increases in morbidity might instead be due to changes in survey questions as well as better reporting practices.

Recently, Manton and colleagues have presented evidence of significant declines in incidences of 16 medical conditions between 1982 and 1989 in persons over age 65. Overall, 11 of 16 conditions showed a decline over the period, with a significant 11 percent reduction in number of conditions per person.

Disability

The condition of disability is of more than semantic importance, because several previous measures of population health status combining mortality and morbidity have focused on disability alone as the morbidity component. In health care this tends to be thought of in terms of conditions or illnesses that limit the ability to satisfactorily perform activities of daily living. The Americans with Disabilities Act of 1990 defined disability as a physical or mental impairment that substantially limits one or more of the major life activities.

Verbrugge indicates that disability is the gap between the body's capability and the environment's demand; she also advocates including in this concept the two less common perspectives of unmet needs and loss of autonomy. Statistical measures of disability have commonly included the number of restricted activity and bed days and the number of persons with long-term limitations of activity due to chronic illness. Since 1982, the National Long Term Care Survey (NLTCS) has measured activities of daily living (ADLs) and instrumental activities of daily living (IADLs).

Disability rates for the elderly fell dramatically from 1989 to 1994, prompting speculation that future Medicare expenditures for the elderly might not increase as dramatically as projected.

Another approach that goes beyond mortality is to consider the quality of life directly. The term quality carries a definition of relating to the degree of excellence and in the health status field is often used generically with regard to the excellence of life years. The boundary between health-related quality of life and health and function is not crisp, but a generally accepted definition is that of various aspects of a person's life which are strongly affected by changes in health status and which encompass dimensions such as generic and condition specific symptoms as well as physical, social, role, and sexual functioning, and mental health.

There is significant concern about the relative usefulness of individual disease-specific measures, in contrast to more generic summary measures of outcome. Many individual disease-specific measures are available. Some argue that only multiple measures at a disease-specific level are appropriate (such as deaths from HIV or severity of depression), because only such specificity allows accurate measurement of health-related quality of life.

Such disease-specific measures are important and valuable for clinicians and programmes working with specifically identified disease groups such as those with AIDS or mental illness or with patients with multiple chronic illnesses, either measuring improvements or lower rates of decline than are expected in many such diseases. However, such disease-specific measures have limitations when one attempts to compare outcomes across different populations and different programmes, since assessing the relative importance of improvement or decline in each measure is difficult, if not impossible.

There has recently been increased interest in measures of quality of care, partly from an academic perspective but largely from the need to provide employers and individuals some standard of quality for health plans and managed care organisations to facilitate informed choices among them. Some of these measures have been developed by individual plans and for Medicare and Medicaid patients.

The US National Committee for Quality Assurance (NCQA) has established a performance measurement programme, the Health Plan Employer Data and Information Set (HEDIS), on which health plans voluntarily report and which purchasers are encouraged to use in judging plan quality. The HEDIS system requires data on a variety of measures in the clinical arena as well as in the areas of access, patient satisfaction, and financial performance. The data set also includes other measures in such areas as access, satisfaction, health plan stability, cost of care, informed choices, and descriptive information.

In addition, this new version also includes a set of testing measures that will be collected on an experimental or trial basis. Examples are persons who smoke, depression treatment continuation, follow-up after Pap smear or mammogram and so on. Such measures have a high degree of face validity and can be of great value for certain purposes; obviously, having higher immunisation rates is better than having lower ones. Programme indicators such as eye care for diabetics are very important data in a diabetic clinic.

Most of these measures do not meet the criteria for outcome measures presented earlier. Having high rates of Pap smears does not guarantee that they are read properly, that positive results are referred to treatment, that any indicated surgery is done promptly and with high quality, and that the net result is longer years of life at maximum levels of quality.

Similarly, additional measures not shown such as high levels of customer satisfaction can be affected by factors that may be desirable, such as pleasant staff and facilities, but that do not necessarily mean that the patients will have longer and/or higher quality lives. Much work by NCQA, FACCT, and other groups is being devoted to developing more sophisticated outcome components for report card measures like HEDIS. But so far these are not sufficient to determine if the overall goal of getting the most health for our health investments has been met.

Such report card measures can help identify health plans that are either outstanding or seriously substandard, but will never be comprehensive and will never be able to guarantee that important aspects of a health plan's quality of care have not deteriorated. It is essential that we develop a better summary measure of length and quality of life for use in purchasing population health, one that accurately reflects outcomes of large enrolled populations or communities.

In terms of measuring improvement in health adjusted life expectancy for an entire population, combining individual measures into an overall composite not only requires that many measures be collected and reported but also necessitates some weighing of each measure into the composite index. The advantage of a single aggregate measure or indicator is that it would allow accurate assessment of comparative baselines as well as changes across different populations. Having a common measure of benefit is essential when comparing alternative financial investments in a cost benefit framework.

There are now several potential approaches for a single measure of health adjusted life expectancy (HALE) that allow the aggregate assessment of population morbidity and mortality together. The first method is that of the quality adjusted life year (QALY), which emphasises the patient's valuation of health status as the quality modifier of life expectancy. Following early work in the United States and England, this method was further elaborated by Torrance, who described the basic concept as quite simple utilities and cardinal values that are assigned to each health state on a scale that is established by assigning a value of 1.0 to being healthy and 0 to being dead.

The utility values reflect the quality of the health states and allow morbidity and mortality improvements to be combined into a single weighted measure, quality adjusted life years (QALYs) gained. Individual QALYs are calculated by multiplying the number of life years expected by the quality adjustment factor derived from patient valuation studies. In the EuroQol rating scale, for example, patients are asked to value their own health state by choosing from three responses in each of five categories: mobility, self-care, usual activities, pain/discomfort, and anxiety/depression. This results in 243 possible combinations of health states, to which have been added unconsciousness and death.

Individual valuations of these states are determined using a visual thermometer scale, where an individual places his or her own health state on a 0 to 100 scale from worst imaginable to best imaginable. The patient's own valuations can then be used to make adjustments of expected life years in different states for alternative treatments or programmes for medical management vs. surgery in patients with severe angina and left main vessel coronary artery disease.

Another measure under active development is that of disability adjusted life years (DALY). Much initial work focused on the combination of mortality and disability, primarily because of the existence and increased quality of survey data of disability measures. Disability is related to morbidity and refers specifically to reduced function in a variety of domains. An early example of this approach was that of Katz and colleagues, who used activity of daily living data from a sample of non-institutionalised people in Massachusetts to determine a measure of active life expectancy.

More recently, Murray has reported on the development of the DALY as, a new indicator of the burden of disease, which uses experts to provide relative weights for a 50 percent reduction in six classes of activity limitation. A generic concern about disability approaches is that they appear to be burden of disease influenced and do not take into account morbidity that does not lead to serious loss of physical function or that occurs outside the physiologic or medical model realm. For example, the DALYs proposed by Murray require more than 50 per cent reduction in function to be counted. On the other hand, they are constructed in large part using data that exists or is being collected in a growing number of population health surveys.

Another important approach is that of years of healthy life (YHL) from Erickson and colleagues. This measure combines two questions already asked in the *US National Health Interview Survey*, one from the disability activity limitation category as well as one regarding general perception of health. This second addition takes the YHL measure beyond the more narrow disability only (DALY) approach critiqued previously. These two questions create a matrix of 30 combinations, to which utility values are assigned that range from 1.00 for persons with excellent health to 0.10 for persons limited in function and in poor health.

These valuations are then applied to age cohorts to create a combination HALE that the researchers call years of healthy life. The advantage of this measure is that it combines disability data with self-reported health status, creating a measure that is available from survey data and represents individual value, but it does so by extrapolating from existing data without doing individual patient surveys as in the EuroQol approach.

Mortality alone is an incomplete measure of health outcome. When these life years are multiplied by a morbidity or quality adjustment factor for each age interval, the result is years of healthy life. A compelling case can be made for such an aggregate measure of health outcome to guide purchasing considerations for moderate to large managed care plans and communities. This does not exclude the usefulness of additional disease-specific measures for individual clinical settings and programmes and for process measures like HEDIS to identify priority areas for improvement.

However, without such a broad and relatively simple measure of health outcome it will be impossible to compare fairly the wide variety of plans and systems for macro financing purposes. The only alternative would be a massive index of hundreds of smaller outcome and process components, with agreed upon weights for each component of the index. This would be a very complicated analytic task and even if possible would be difficult to explain. With health adjusted life expectancy adopted as the conceptual measure of health outcome for the purpose of purchasing population health, it is both possible and advantageous to quickly but carefully move to an aggregate measure such as years of healthy life as the specific measurement tool for a health outcome incentive standard.

The efficacy of many health care practices is unknown, that one-dimensional measurement strategies may miss underlying multiple and independent attributes of health, that process characteristics such as respect and caring have value, and that evaluation can detect flaws in design or process even if a defective product has not yet been produced downstream.

Smith has described a series of unintended consequences of managing to performance indicators and suggests strategies for dealing with them. Similarly, Heather Palmer has indicated that issues such as patient preferences, unknown risk factors, sample size, time for outcomes to be observed, and error in patient reported outcomes pose difficulties for outcome measurements; she indicates her preference for disease-specific guideline performance measures. It is legitimate to ask whether process measures such as satisfaction or provider compassion or quality of facilities should be given weight in a purchasing population health framework. It cannot be denied that these are important considerations to almost everyone and in addition have economic value.

It might be useful to separate such process components measures into three categories with regard to their impact on health outcomes. First, some process factors such as peace of mind or compliance with medication routine, which actually contribute to the healing process, are at least theoretically incorporated into this framework, since positive outcomes will be increased. In the second category it is likely that there are some aspects of care that may actually reduce positive outcomes, such as the charming but unqualified surgeon or procedures that are harmful. Even if such things are desired by patients, there is no rationale for encouraging them, and they probably should be eliminated through whatever mechanism is effective. This leaves us with the third intermediate category of process components that may be desired by patients or providers but neither help nor hurt outcome.

How these should be valued is less clear, although they ought to be judged luxuries, available to those who want to use their own resources to acquire them. Some persons consider them very important: a recent study revealed that a significant fraction of patients in a Scottish infertility clinic would have preferred not to become pregnant if staff attitudes were not satisfactory. Public resources should not be used for such beyond outcome investments while measurable outcome improvement is still possible for other patients. It is also possible in a competitive system that such issues will be dealt with in part through patient choice of health plans. Such concerns and process considerations must be accommodated in a Purchasing Population Health framework.

But in the absence of an ultimate outcome standard such as health adjusted life expectancy, a tyranny of process can and does become an end in itself. More than a few organisations have invested much time and resources in managerial processes such as corporate restructuring and/or quality improvement, with little demonstrated benefit to patients in terms of ultimate health outcomes. There is still much uncertainty regarding what is effective in producing population health, and this is likely to continue for some time, if not forever. For those interventions that are relatively clear, professional guidelines such as those advocated by Palmer will be adopted by organisations at the patient care level and built into professional practice and reward structures.

But for many less certain interventions, a global incentive at the integrated organisational level will encourage profe-ssional and administrative creativity to identify additional interventions that are most cost-effective in produ-cing the desired outcome for the whole population. As opposed to our being continually locked into incentives that reward only for providing additional medical services and increased revenues, the HALE purchasing population health outcome framework will lead to scores of natural efforts and experiments to find medical and health interventions that will produce units of outcome improvement at the lowest marginal cost.

TRENDS IN HEALTH EXPENDITURES

Health care in our country accounts for one-seventh of our national economy, and it includes institutions and services that are of critical, often life and death, importance to the population. Many depend on the health care industry for jobs; one person's health expenditure is another's income. In many areas, both rural and urban, health care employment is critical to the economy of the area. For most individuals the system works, even though increasing numbers of people are calling for change because of insecurity about coverage or worry about costs.

Changing the system by increasing coverage and/or decreasing costs requires a clear and compelling rationale or it will be met with resistance by patients and providers who are sceptical of change. To build outcomes into fundamental managerial and financial incentive structures, a health outcome purchasing standard is essential. The costs of health care are high and increasing. We have all experienced the high price of hospital care, emergency room visits, medications, and nursing home care, whether or not insurance is available. We also know this because in the mid-1980s a public policy debate surfaced that focused attention on these costs over the past two decades. State and federal legislators were looking at automatic increases in public spending for Medicaid and Medicare created by price and volume increases, and employers were facing the growth in fringe benefit costs.

Keeping track of national health expenditures is complex, primarily because of the pluralistic nature of our system and the many different cost and revenue centres that it encompasses. This is relatively easy for public programmes like Medicare and Medicaid where national and state figures are available. It is not so straightforward for non-governmental expenditures through private insurance or out-of-pocket cash payments, since no such comparable central data source exists.

In US, for hospital care, data is obtained from the American Hospital Association survey of hospital revenues. For physician and dentist expenses, a sample of tax records from the Internal Revenue Service is used. Combining data from multiple sources, an annual report is produced by the Office of the Actuary of the Health Care Financing Administration.

Costs can either be shown as total dollars or as per capita expenditures, but such numbers need to be adjusted for the overall price increases in the economy from inflation. It has become common for comparative purposes across time and across countries to report expenditures as a per cent of the total gross domestic product, which incorporates the inflation factor.

In US, Annual increases in the medical care component of the Consumer Price Index (CPT) have approached the general inflation rate for the first time since the late 1970s. This trend recently prompted the Medicare Prospective Payment Assessment Commission to recommend for the first time ever that Congress not increase payment rates to hospitals in 1997. However, at the same time, some employer benefits consultants began to advise in early 1997 that recent slowdowns are only temporary and that high single digit or even double digit increases are increasingly possible in 1998 and beyond.

While data comparability is an issue when crossing national expenditure systems, expenditures reported from the 13 developed countries in the Office of European Cooperation and Development are similar enough for accurate gross comparison. While almost all countries are experiencing growth, the United States leads the world both in per capita expenditures and in recent growth.

In 1993 there was a twofold difference in total per capita expenditures across the states. Of course, states differ in characteristics such as wage rates, number of elderly, and number of persons who come into the state for expensive care. However, one analysis showed that these demographic factors accounted for only about one-third of the variation, with the remainder associated with other characteristics of the state health care environment such as the numbers of physicians and hospital beds.

During 1970-80, economy-wide inflation dominated the picture, since 1980 medical care price inflation was very significant, as was the large increase in intensity in 1990-91. When these rates of increase over general inflation rates continue, the per cent of GDP devoted to health expenditures increases automatically. Specific factors for the increase include the following: rising physician incomes, an excess of specialists, the aging of the population, paperwork and administration, defensive medicine in the malpractice climate, and new technology. All of these and more play a role.

In the United States we are using more services than are effective in improving our overall health status. A recent study comparing Canadian and US physician expenditures indicated that Canadians received a higher volume of services for lower total expenditures, explained entirely by lower physician fees. Within the United States, the pioneering work of John Wennberg has pointed out the significant variation in the number of medical and surgical procedures, such as hysterectomies, in different areas of the country, even after correcting for underlying differences in illness rates

An increasing number of studies are showing the extent of inappropriate or unnecessary care. The current practice of medicine is far from perfect. One-fourth of hospital deaths may be preventable, and one-third of some hospital procedures may expose patients to risk without improving their health. One-third of drugs may not be indicated, and one-third of abnormal laboratory tests may not be followed up by physicians. While considerable research and clinical attention are focusing on finding these variations and correcting any inappropriate medical interventions, the absence of clear health outcome measures limits the effectiveness of traditional economic forces in achieving this goal.

There are several reasons for the so-called market failure in health care, but the main one of relevance here is the lack of perfect information between customer and seller. Someone buying a car can obtain fairly complete information about the product from inspection, advertising, consumer magazines, and a test drive. Even repair records from past years' models are available, and good information about reasonable prices exists. The main reason for the difference in health care is the complex and scientific nature of medicine.

Much of modern medicine is rooted in basic scientific principles that are not easily understood by those without appropriate training. Indeed, some aspects of complex drugs and procedures are not completely understood by physicians of another specialty. Currently there are major advances in the amount of information available to consumers, increasingly in the electronic interactive form.

Although the role of the patient in his or her own health outcome improvement has increased, it has not yet become a significant force in the marketplace. Furthermore, much of medicine remains an art, in that precise rules and guidelines in many situations are neither available nor possible. For instance, one of the reasons for the variations in the number of surgical procedures in different regions of the United States is that there is a zone of uncertainty in many cases where clear indications do not exist and professional judgement necessarily takes over. Another reason that market forces do not fully apply to medical care is that patients often do not want to be involved in the evaluation of their doctor or hospital in the same way they would when buying a new car or a brand of beer.

Health care is personal and often of life and death importance, and the belief that someone else is in charge and knows best is frequently desired. This is reflected in survey results over time that indicate that Americans are critical of the health care system but not of their own providers. This is changing to some degree with better patient education materials and even interactive computer programmes that allow patients to learn about their options and to indicate their preferences, particularly in areas of professional uncertainty. But to the extent that clear information to evaluate outcomes of medical care exists at all, it remains largely in the professional domain.

Another major reason for the lack of influence of market forces is that health care professionals and institutions have not had either the tools or the incentives to develop outcome standards at the population level themselves. This statement is in no way intended to demean the intentions and motivations of health care clinicians and managers. With rare exceptions they are trained and committed to both high quality care and positive outcomes for their patients, and of course obtaining good outcomes at the individual clinical procedure level is commonplace. But data about what has worked for many different patients over time in varied, complex circumstances is not routinely available, and memory and anecdote are imperfect.

New computer technology will aid in this in the future, but in many cases outcome information simply does not exist, and often long-term follow-up is not possible. For many years, financial incentives have favoured doing more rather than less, since under a fee-for-service system each additional visit test or operation yields additional income to the clinician and/ or institution. It is not surprising that physicians and hospitals behave a rational economic actors, providing more and more services, particularly in areas of professional uncertainty. However, both regulatory and market based reform have begun to reverse these fee-for-service incentives. For hospital payment, Medicare reforms in 1984 introduced the Prospective Payment System, which pays hospitals for an entire admission rather than for each day of a hospital stay.

This system created more than 400 Diagnostic Related Groups (DRGs), which bundled all days and tests for each category of treatment into a single standard rate and created incentives for fewer days as well as for looking carefully at the tests and other services provided during the admission in business terms, this would be the equivalent of a fixed price contract instead of a cost plus contract. But while DRG payments began to control costs within a hospital stay, they did nothing to control the number of admissions themselves. They also led to increased expenditures outside of the hospital such as for home care services.

The advent of managed care takes such incentives another step, bringing both the volume and the price of services under scrutiny. Under managed care arrangements, doctors and hospitals in a coordinated system agree to provide all needed care to a group of employees or Medicare or Medicaid recipients for a specified rate per person for a fixed period of time, usually a year. Managed care replaces the economic pressure for overutilisation in fee for service with incentives to reduce utilisation.

While early growth was in the employer based insurance markets, currently 32 per cent of Medicaid and 10 per cent of Medicare recipients are enrolled in managed care plans. There are a large variety of such plans, ranging from not-for-profit tightly managed group-staff models to for profit loosely formed networks of physicians and hospitals, often run by agreements.

Even powerful managed care incentives have not dealt fully with the cost-containment issue for several reasons. The first is that even at 4 per cent real growth, the share of GDP devoted to health care will continue to rise, if at a slower rate. It is unclear whether it is realistic to expect that the percent of GDP devoted to health can actually fall, although we have seen examples of other nations that have much lower levels of national resources devoted to health care. Beyond the problem of actually reducing health expenditures as a percentage of GDP, there is the additional difficulty that many persons are still not in managed care systems or other types of systems that coordinate care more efficiently. Also, cost reductions are achieved not only by eliminating unnecessary services but also by decreasing benefits and/or by increasing co-payments to the patient for certain services such as medications and ambulatory visits. While this may lower the premiums that employers have to pay the managed care plans, it does not necessarily lower expenditures either to the individual or to the nation.

Furthermore, in many managed care plans, only hospital and physician services are covered, leaving many components of health care outside the system. Finally, in many markets, competition between plans has led to duplication of equipment, facilities, specialists, and advertising in order to attract and keep patients in a particular plan. But whatever the current limitations, it is generally agreed that economic incentives such as DRGs and managed care, which require providers and insurers to carefully examine their services and costs, have great potential for savings in the long run, certainly in comparison to the undisciplined fee-for-service incentives that are in large part responsible for the growth in health expenditures already described.

The best evidence about the relationship between health status and health expenditures comes from international comparisons of health expenditures and mortality rates. There has long been a positive relationship between life expectancy and national per capita income but that a decreasing return begins to develop at higher expenditure levels. Diminishing marginal return is an important concept both in economics and in population health; it refers to lower increases in output for equivalent additional increases in input. Without formal analysis it is not difficult to accept the likelihood that investments in pure water and immunisations will greatly improve health status in very poor countries, while more complex and costly investments in medical care, prevention, and the environment are probably necessary for health outcome improvement in the developed world .

Mortality alone is a limited measure of health, and there is a paucity of data going beyond this measure. In the United States, every year the Northwestern National Life Insurance Company releases its profile of the relative health of the 50 states. Their measure of health is a weighted composite of 19 factors, including mortality from several causes. Although this index requires validation by other researchers, it is usually picked up by national newspapers and is clearly in the public domain.

There is a correct level of health expenditure as a percentage of GDP or some other economic or health care indicator. But the amount of resources involved in US health expenditures at the flat of the curve is enormous. There is an opportunity to reduce the rate of growth in health expenditures, and even the absolute level over time, yielding savings for which a country with limited resources could find productive use, either in health care or in other sectors.

There have been beginning discussions about making a twenty-first century paradigm shift to redefine the product of the health care system as population health status, and to create economic incentives in these integrated health care delivery systems and other health promoting sectors of society to produce health in the most cost-effective manner. A purchasing population health framework would encourage the establishment of outcomes for each community or health plan;

the goal would be to decrease mortality, morbidity, and disability as efficiently as possible. In such a system, explicit financial incentives would be developed to ensure movement toward improvement of the health status of populations. Such a focus would turn attention to outcomes rather than structure or process and would unleash forces that would capture the attention of health providers, health institutions, and other health enhancing sectors of society.

It should reassure those concerned about managed care incentives for underutilisation and skimming of profits, since agreed upon and accountable measures of performance would be in place; if for-profit plans could deliver equal or better risk adjusted outcomes than non-profit or public providers and still return profit to shareholders, this policy concern might vanish. It would also stimulate a wide array of creative approaches to begin to make progress toward this new goal.

REFERENCES

Afifi, A. and Breslow L., 1994, 'The Maturing Paradigm of Public Health', *Annu.Rev.Pub.Health*, 15:223-35.

Evans R., Hodge M. and Press I., 1994, 'Why are Some People Healthy and Others not?':, *The Determinants of Health of Populations*, New York, Adine de Gruyter.

House J.S., Landis K and Umberson D., 1988, 'Social Relationship and Health, *Science* 241:540-45.

Institute of Medicine, 1988, *The Future of Public Health*, New York, DC: National Academy Press.

Bibliography

Berg, F., 'Nondiet movement gains strength', *Obesity and Health* 6:85-90, 1992.

Bowen, D.J. et al., 'Influences on eating patterns of change to a lowfat diet, *JADA* 93:1309-1311, 1993.

Bradford N. Strand Ed Scantling Martin Johnson, *Fitness Education: Teaching Concepts-Based Fitness in the Schools*, 1997.

Brian Luke Seaward, *Health of the Human Spirit: Spiritual Dimensions for Personal Health*, 2001.

Bud Getchell Alan E. Mikesky Kay Mikesky, *Physical Fitness: A Way of Life*, 1998.

Carrier, K., M. Steinhardt, and S. Bowman, 'Rethinking traditional weight management programs: A 3-year follow-up evaluation of a new approach', *Journal of Psychology* 128: 517535, 1994.

Cooper, Robert K., *Health And Fitness Excellence*, Boston: Houghton Mifflin, 1989.

Daniel Girdano, Dorothy E. Dusek George S. Everly, *Controlling Stress and Tension*, 2001.

Darden, Ellington, *Living Longer Stronger*, New York: Burkley Publishing, 1995.

David K. Miller T. Earl Allen, *Fitness: A Lifetime Commitment*, 1995.

Dr.Krishna Raman, *A Matter of Health: Intergration of Yoga and Western Meidcine to Prevention and Care*, 1998, Eastwest Books, Madras.

Edwards, Sally, *Sally Edwards' Heart Zone Training: Exercise Smart, Stay Fit, And Live Longer*, Holbrook, MA: Adams Publishing, 1996.

Fletcher, Anne, *Thin for Life*, Shelburne, VT: Chapters Publishing, 1994.

Foreyt, J.P. and G. K. Goodrick, 'Weight management without dieting', *Nutrition Today* 28 (2): 4-9, 1993.

Hoeger, Werner and Sharon Hoeger, *Lifetime Physical Fitness And Wellness*, Englewood, CO: Morton Publishing, 1992.

James F. McKenzie Jan L. Smeltzer, *Planning, Implementing, and Evaluating Health Promotion Programs: A Primer*, 2001.

James J. Neutens Laurna Rubinson, *Research Techniques for the Health Sciences*, 1997.

Jan Galen Bishop *Fitness Through Aerobics,* 1999.

Jerold S. Greenberg George S. DintimanBarbee Myers Oakes, *Physical Fitness and Wellness*, 1998.

Jerrold S. Greenberg George B. Dintiman Barbee Myers Oakes, *Wellness: Creating a Life of Health and Fitness*, 1997.

John A. Romas M.P.H., Ph.D. Manoj Sharma M.B.B.S., Ph.D., *Practical Stress Management: A Comprehensive Workbook for Managing Change and Promoting Health*, 2000.

Joseph W. Donnelly Norm Eburne Mark Kittleson, *Mental Health: Dimensions of Self-Esteem and Emotional Well-Being*, 2001.

Kingsbury, B., *Full Figure Fitness: A Program for Teaching Overweight Adults*, Champaign, IL: Life Enhancement Publications, 1993.

Kirkley, George and John Goodbody, *The Manual of Weight Training*, London: Stanley Paul, 1994.

Larry Brown, H., *Lifetime Fitness*, 1996.

McGuigan, F.J., *Encyclopedia of Stress,* 1999.

Noril, Christopher, *The Weight Training Principles and Practice Manual*, London: A & C Publishing, 1993.

Obesity (Lucent Overview Series), Akers, Charlene Library binding, ISBN: 1560066628.

Obesity: Pathophysiology, Psychology, and Treatment, (Chapman and Hall Series in Clinical Nutrition), Blackburn, George L. Kanders, Beatrice S. (eds.) Hardcover ISBN: 041298461X.

Obvious Guide To Medical Survival, Thomas, Frank M., Jr. Paperback ISBN: 0970632606.

Occupational Disease in Relation to Compensation and Health Insurance (Columbia University, Studies in the Social Sciences, No 345), Goldberg, Rosamond W., Hardcover ISBN: 040451345X.

Occupational Health Nursing Care Guidelines, Daly-Gawenda, Debra (eds.), Hudson, Edsel K. (eds.), Perea, Carol (ed.), Paperback, ISBN: 0826193501.

Oil That Heals: A Physicians Successes With Caster Oil Treatments, Mcgarey, William A., Paperback, ISBN: 0876043082.

Oil-Protein Diet Cookbook, Budwig, Johanna, Paperback, ISBN: 0969527225.

Omega 3 Oils, Rudin, Donald Paperback, ISBN: 0895297213.

Omega Diet, Wills, Judith Paperback, ISBN: 074727195X.

Omega Diet: The Lifesaving Nutritional Program Based On The Diet Of The Island Of Crete, Simopoulos, Artemis P., Paperback, ISBN: 0060930233.

Omichinski, Linda and Kathleen Harrison,'Nondiet Weight Management: A Lifestyle Approach to Health and Fitness', San Marcos, *Nutrition Dimension,* 1995.

Omichinski, Linda, 'A paradigm shift from weight loss to healthy living', *Obesity and Health* 7:48-50, 1993.

On The Run: Exercise And Fitness For Busy People, Waitz, Grete, Paperback, ISBN: 1579542530.

Optimum Health For The New Millennium, Townsend, Ernestine Paperback ISBN: 0738837970.

Optimum Nutrition, Holford, Patrick Paperback ISBN: 1870976053.

Organic Living, Van Straten, Michael Hardcover/Clothcover ISBN: 0875969305.

Patricia A. Reagan Jodi Brookins Fisher, *Community Health in the 21st Century*, 1997.

Peterson, James, Cedric Bryant and Susan Peterson, 'Strength Training for Women', Champaign, IL; Human Kinetics, 1992.

Randall R. Cottrell James T. Girvan James F. McKenzie, *Principles and Foundations of Health Promotion and Education*, 1999

Rebecca J. Donatelle Lorraine G. Davis, *Access to Health*, 2000.

_______________ , *Health: The Basics,* 2001.

Richard Polidoro J., *Sport and Physical Activity in the Modern World*, 2000.

Robert W. Buckingham Ph.D., *Primer on International Health*, 2001.

Sally A. Althoff Milan Svoboda Daniel Girdano, *Choices in Wellness for Life*, 1996.

Scharzenegger, Arnold, *The Encyclopedia of Modern Bodybuilding*, New York: Simon & Schuster, 1987.

Scott K. Powers Stephen L. Dodd, *Total Fitness: Exercise, Nutrition, and Wellness*, 1999.

Sharon A. Plowman Denise L. Smith, *Exercise Physiology: For Health, Fitness and Performance*, 1997.

Terry J. Housh Ph.D. Dona J. Housh Ph.D., *Introduction to Exercise Science*, 2000.

Thomas D. Fahey Ed.D., *Super Fitness for Sports, Conditioning, and Health*, 2000.

Weider, Joe and Bill Reynolds, *Ultimate Bodybuilding*, Chicago: Contemporary Books, 1989.

William F. Stier, *Managing Sport, Fitness, and Recreation Programs: Concepts and Practices*, 1999.

Index